FROM FAMILY TO FACTORY

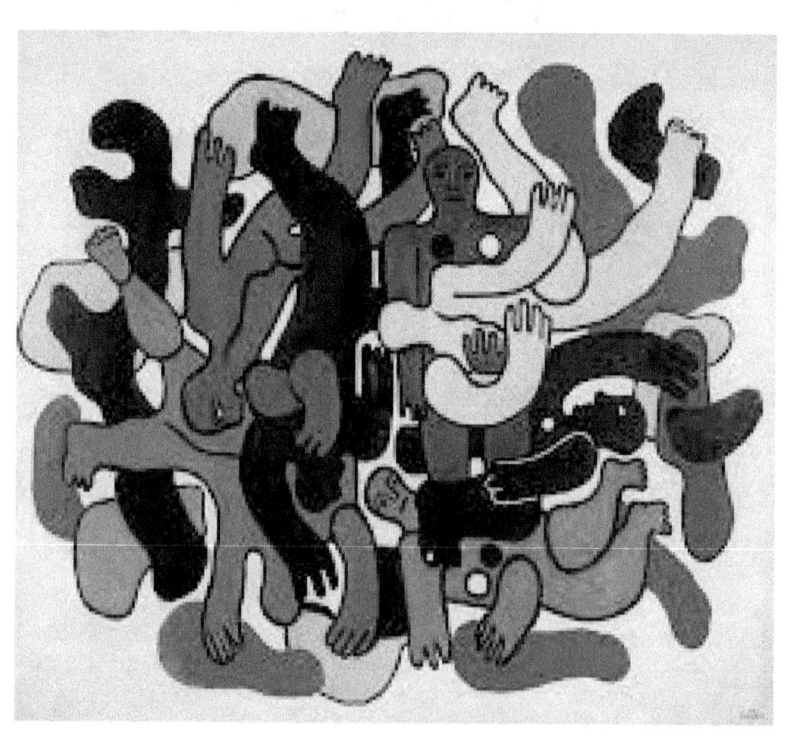

FROM FAMILY TO FACTORY

Lost personal meaning in healthcare

Essays 2004 - 2014

Volume 2:
If you want good personal Healthcare
See a Vet

DAVID ZIGMOND

Printed by CreateSpace

ISBN-13: 978-1515016915
ISBN-10: 1515016919

Contents

Introduction

This is the second of three volumes of writings about the more humanly complex aspects of our healthcare. Although sequential and complementary, each of the three volumes can be read alone. The combined anthology is published as *If You Want Good Personal Healthcare, See a Vet*. Volume One contains additional historical and introductory comment.

From Family to Factory compiles more recent articles. These have been written as a reaction: spurred by my witnessing an ever-rising tide of depersonalisation in the healthcare system that has long employed me and will eventually care for me. I have seen that as the technology becomes better, our shared human connection and understanding has often become worse.

A decade ago my voice was more solitary. More recently, especially since several debacles epitomised by Mid Staffs, there are many more consternated voices calling for human reconnection.

What has gone wrong? These writings offer several seminal notions. For example: that the dramatic successes of the biomechanical model has then led to its harmful excesses; that indiscriminate use of language and thought – of the type that seeks to control, define or manipulate – will displace other forms of consciousness and engagement; that the volume of electronic signalling is inversely proportional to the quality of personal contact and communication; that excessive preoccupation with the measurable often leads to hazardous neglect of what is not; that unless we are very careful, our push-buttoned world leads us into a Virtual Realm where we are all liable to the agitated disconnections of ADHD.

Such emerging notions have led me to a guiding maxim about our work: *Healthcare is a humanity guided by science. That humanity is an art and an ethos.* Yes, our science is bigger and better – but what has happened to our art and ethos in healthcare? And what are the consequences?

These decade-spanned articles are my answers to those questions. They draw from my frontline work as a doctor in a culture where the human need is growing, but the human responsiveness is shrinking. I illustrate all this with many stories of patients, doctors and various cohorts: they are all conventionally disguised, but kept as veracious as I am able.

A long, critical Glossary is offered for interested readers who are not familiar with some of the institutional and organisational terms.

David Zigmond, August 2015

Glossary of Institutional Terms

Much of the writing of this Volume encounters our increasing and severe healthcare conundrae: these are largely consequent to our over-industrialisation of the Medical Model. This has become particularly clear in the cultural and political turmoil besetting Britain's National Health Service.

The interest and importance of these issues extends far beyond this already vast arena, but the organisational events are very complex and often difficult to understand: examples may need explanation. This is even more likely for readers who are not healthcare workers or British residents. As a bridge to clarity and comprehension, I have constructed this critical glossary of key terms. Many of the italicised words are cross-referenced: this helps to give an outline of the current System's skeleton. Some key terms are worth highlighting but are widely known and understood: for economy of space I have italicised but not glossaried these.

Algorithm. A templated and flow-charted system of defined and logical steps prescribed to analyse and manage identified problems. Can be readily diagrammed and computerised. Has rapid appeal due to its standardised reproducibility, apparent clarity, precision and logic. Disadvantages: deals poorly with real-life's ambiguity, variation, meaning and complexity. Can displace individually responsive and intelligent judgement and imagination.

Appraisals for healthcare staff. A formal procedure whose purpose is to monitor and assure quality and safety of professional performance and development. Much effort has been made to standardise and, when possible, quantify such complex evaluations. Guidance has been sought from the newer professions of business management and consultancy. The aspiration is far less controvertible than the results: for the formalistic segues easily to the formulaic. Subsequent attempts to make procedure 'fair and comprehensive' commonly become burdensome, blind and bureaucratic. Generally professionals have described their experiences of appraisals as elaborate rituals of proffered compliance and verbalised obedience. Far fewer report the kind of intelligent searching dialogue that will helpfully identify or clarify important problems.

Balint. Michael Balint (1896-1970) was a psychoanalyst who, in the 1950s and 1960s, explored the 'subtext' of medical consultations. He started with a small group of London GPs, but his influence expanded to galvanise a generation of doctors to think about inexplicit meaning, encoded actions and attachments, and the possibility of both treatment and illness as kinds of preverbal or paraverbal language. Many GPs experienced their work as enriched and enlightened by such informal and qualitative research. This brief, rich flowering was largely extinguished by the rapid rise of systems that demanded quantification, standardised codes, and mass-reproducibility.

Evidence Based Medicine has great difficulty accommodating Balint's subtle invitations to explore meaning.

Care Quality Commission (CQC). A governmental network of healthcare inspectors. This is similar in mission to the *Appraisal* of professional individuals, but applied to the healthcare organisation that employs them. As with Appraisals, the task is certainly necessary and important but its sensible and accurate execution very difficult. Again, presentations of formulaic compliance can easily mask deeper lack of integrity. The shocking debacle at *Mid Staffs* examples what can be missed by 'competent' yet routinised methods of inspection.

Clinical Commissioning Group (CCG). A recently mandated executive network for deciding, defining, procuring and purchasing the healthcare needs of an allocated geographical population. The boards are now dominated by local GPs but contain other healthcare professionals and lay members. The CCG has replaced the *Primary Care Trust (PCT)*, which was administered, ultimately, by non-clinical managers.

The aspiration – for democratic healthcare decisions that are locally responsive and responsible, and professionally decided – seems laudable. The unravelling reality is less so: multitasking, overmanaged and weary GPs already have much diminished time for their traditional role as personal physicians and cannot give adequate, good attention to this new and very complex task. The result is an expedient short-circuiting to a hastily assembled (and thus often not competent) network of oligarchies that are themselves likely to be in thrall to a very flawed *Internal Market*.

Cognitive Behaviour Therapy (CBT). An attempt to schematise and standardise therapeutic psychological contact for the mentally or behaviourally troubled. It is largely based on depersonalised diagnostic categories, focused on the symptomatic and explicit, and guided by *algorithms* and *Care*

Pathways. It is readily (if speciously) computer-coded and measurable: CBT thus has appeal to planners, economists, managers and the kinds of practitioners who share their mindset. The limitations are similar to all algorithms and Care Pathways: the model has difficulty with complexity, variation, meaning and imagination – and thus can easily impoverish practitioners' personal resources to deal with these.

Commissioning. A currently common term for design, negotiation and procurement of services within the marketised NHS. Like other devices to industrialise and monetarise healthcare it is least problematic when applied to healthcare problems that are generally resolved rapidly and reliably by standardised technical procedure (eg hip replacements). *Pastoral Healthcare* (eg psychiatry) starkly exposes its limitations.

Commodification. The attempt to treat and process all healthcare activities as if they are manufactured objects or geophysical resources. This can work relatively well in tasks that have clear and stable boundaries. *Pastoral Healthcare*, by contrast, needs vocational and holistic attitudes that cannot be processed in this way. Nevertheless, commodification makes welcome sense to planners and managers in conducting many aspects of the *Internal Market*. Experiences from frontline health workers are far less tidy: for many years there have been mounting, frustrated expressions of clinical and personal meaninglessness and the stymying of good personal care.

Community Mental Health Team (CMHT). Thirty years ago CMHTs were vaunted as a progressive face of the future, consummated by the closure of the old *Mental Hospitals*. Instead mentally distressed patients would be speedily streamed to community-based specialisms. The specialists themselves professionally progress via certified trainings rather than personal qualities or vocation. Recent healthcare management thinking – much derived from 1980s Japanese car manufacturing – promised more efficient, accessible and responsive help. As elsewhere in the NHS, this attempt to industrialise pastoral healthcare produces results that often become inefficient and perverse.

Evidence-based Medicine (EBM). This has been introduced into healthcare to optimise the reliability and efficiency of therapeutic interventions. The idea is to invest in language and procedures that are officially sanctioned by scientific rigour, and then *Governance*. Healthcare economists and planners favour EBM because it is apparently objective, clear and unambiguous – and can then extirpate the errors and obfuscations of the personal and subjective. In this way *Quantification*, *Standardisation* and *Commodification* are all expedited. EBM thus becomes a key component in the *Internal Market*.

EBM is yet another example from healthcare of how a model's attractive simplicity may be woefully inadequate for complex realities. EBM has mostly operated from evidence restricted to the quantifiable and reproducible. This makes a base that is deemed 'safe', but is also narrow and rigid. It may be necessary, but it often is not sufficient. Problems arise because EBM may be loaded with an authority it cannot bear. Very often the most important aspects of human experience and variation cannot be directly measured or objectified. This is far more than any administrative anomaly: for the unmappable area is the massive – yet vulnerable – human heart of healthcare. EBM, in compatible areas, may be a valuable guiding principle: aggrandised to wider and rigid diktat, it can do real harm.

Increased Access to Psychological Treatment Services (IAPTS). A late parallel, and equivalent, to *CMHTs*. The task focus is therapeutic psychology (not psychiatry). Similar processes are used to identify, stream and manage problems: diagnoses, *Care Pathways* and (especially) the use of *CBT* as a procedural intervention. The system is designed to be easily compatible with electronic informatics, the *Internal Market* and *Payment by Results*. Some also argue that it helps equity and fairness of distribution. The flaws are largely common to those of the *CMHT*.

Internal Market. In the early 1990s this was a seminal and radical idea: to introduce monetarist values and mechanisms to nationalised healthcare. The enormous federal cooperative network would be broken up into economically and occupationally autarkic *NHS Trusts*. Wide and informal affiliations were replaced by a complex system of *Purchaser-Provider Splits*, which need tending by ceaseless negotiations to facilitate 'trade' between the Trusts. Computerised, quantifiable data, *Care Pathways* and *Payment by Results* are all necessary developments to service this Internal Market. The idea is to positively influence motivation and focus attention. After more than twenty years' evolution the results are mixed and highly contentious. Many longer-term observers (myself included) assess the losses as much greater than the gains. Since the recent Health and Social Care Act there is now more possibility of an external market: this amplifies contention.

Mid-Staffs. Refers to the Mid Staffordshire NHS Trust. In recent years perplexed and appalled attention has focused on the clear and massive failures and abuses of care uncovered in this NHS hospital. The widespread institutional human disengagement has been shocking enough. Further grotesquerie is provided by the attractive and respectable public persona of the Trust: it had received very favourable reports from routine official inspections, eg by the *CQC*. Mid Staffs is one of many egregious examples of concealed inhumanities in current NHS healthcare, though the most notorious. Many see Mid Staffs as being a kind of diabolic iconic: a harsh signal of the consequences of abandoning healthcare's primal task of human recognition and connection. Such abandonment, it is argued, is due largely to the rise of the *Internal Market's* 3Cs (Competition, Commissioning and Commodification) and a culture cowed by managed demands for numerous, rigid and narrow *targets* and *PBR*. Subsequent statements from Mid Staffs' employees have described a bullied and intimidated work culture redolent of factory workers a century earlier.

National Institute for Health and Care Excellence (NICE). A governmentally appointed network of experts tasked with evaluating and applying *EBM* in specified areas of healthcare. As its operational nucleus is EBM, it has the same assets, limitations and liabilities. Thus NICE makes its most competent contributions to healthcare problems that are clearly physically defined, and which can then be reliably resolved or contained by standardised physical procedures.

So, NICE-prescribed frameworks usually make good and useful (though not infallible) contributions to the care of, say, Diabetes or Hypertension. Yet this kind of *algorithmic* management fares far less well with the vast human variations of pastoral healthcare (eg mood disturbance or alcoholism) where individual practitioners' wisdom, experience and subtle hues of judgement are central and indispensable.

Pastoral Healthcare. A term little used, but increasingly needed. It refers to our guiding human matrix of care: all those personal influences that comfort, heal, guide, contain, encourage, vitalise and illuminate. Pastoral healthcare thus extends far beyond any procedure or formula. Although certainly including such activities as personally attuned 'mental healthcare' or 'psychotherapy', it is not confined to these. Good Pastoral Healthcare is synonymous with the heart, soul and broader intellect involved throughout our encounters with others' distress. Like so many holistic activities, its subtler enactments cannot be readily measured, coded or proceduralised: Pastoral Healthcare thus tends to be neglected, displaced or destroyed by a culture dominated by the *Internal Market* and such satellite procedures as *Payment by Results, Evidence Based Medicine, Quality Outcome Frameworks* etc.

Payment by Results (PBR). The intention and thinking behind this kind of infusion of commercial motivation is relatively clear. It often galvanises manufacturing industries. Yet the consequences – when applied to complex human welfare – become frequently obscure, tangled and perverse. Results of complex activities are often difficult to define, measure or predict. Motivation in welfare is – and should be – much broader and more complex than that of commerce. Unbridled PBR in healthcare provides specious statistics, bad science and egregiously perverse incentives.

Primary Care Trust (PCT). For several years this body preceded the *CCG* in managing the trade and conduct of Community Practitioners (GPs, Dentists, Pharmacists, District Nurses, Health Visitors, Chiropodists etc). It was managed largely by non-clinicians: the transition to CCGs brings doubtful benefits as few GPs can maintain the long-term personal resources necessary for the complexity and size of the task.

QUOF (Quality Outcomes Framework). A complex system of remuneration for GPs, constituting a kind of 'performance related pay'. This is based on electronically guided and recorded *Specific Performance Indicators,* themselves based on *algorithms* and *Care Pathways* designed by governmental think-tanks and committees. The resultant computerised systems monitor and signal how each practitioner is managing each encounter with a patient with a chronic disease or risk. QUOF has thus brought the government and the computer into the centre of the consulting room in an unprecedented way. The results are mixed. The gains are most clear in bringing more vigilant and systematic management to high risk conditions where therapeutics are clearly effective (eg Hypertension and

Coronary Heart Disease), and detection of some other areas of significant risk/poor engagement. The losses are from displacement. Computer informatics and governmentally dictated tasks replace subtle, personally nuanced exchanges that are essential for comfort, understanding and healing influences. Such undesignated 'softer' activities are also essential to NHS staff morale. The QUOF-directed GP has become more of a public health commissar than a personal physician: patients are increasingly 'efficiently' treated, but poorly understood.

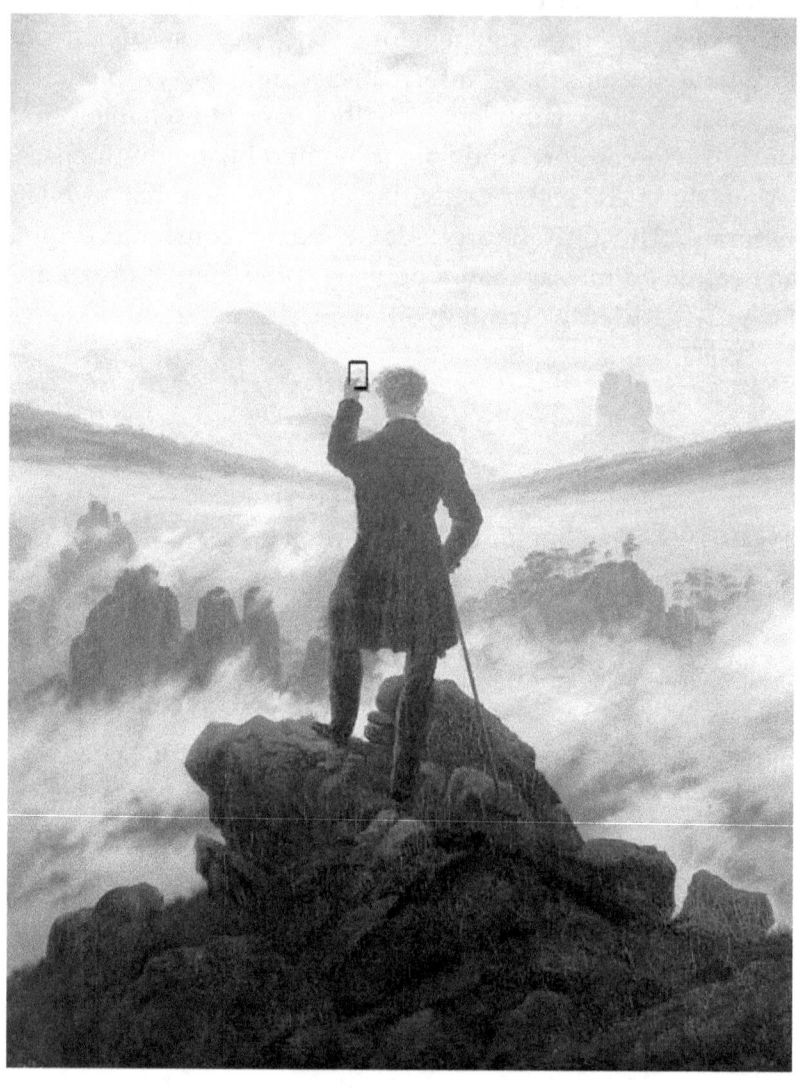

C. D. Friedrich – *The Wanderer above the Mist* 1818
(upgraded 2012)

Where in the World are You?

Miraculous cyber; insidious dislocation

What do mobile communications, internet sex and modern over-schematised mental health systems have in common?
– a computer mediated disconnection of intended content from embedding human context.
What happens?

Introduction

Our increasingly easy and instant access to knowledge and products is usually regarded as 'progress', yet, paradoxically, often deprives us of more organic forms of discovery, connection and creativity. This is a growing problem that we are ingeniously disregarding. Mobile phones, internet sex, Sat Navs and computer-systematised mental healthcare are exampled and explored.

*

'A thing in itself never expresses anything. It is the relation between things that gives meaning to them'

Hans Hofman, *Search for the Real* (1967)

I miss the call. I recognise the number but cannot identify it: I call back. The voice is reassuring in its immediate familiarity; a softly musical, slightly apologetic lilt, a faint West Country burr. It is a voice I have known for many years; it is so clear that I know she must be calling from somewhere close by. Yet she has recently talked of imminent departure for a late-career gap-year; travelling to long-envisioned, little-known, distant places.

I continue to misconstrue: 'Where in the world are you?' I ask, part genuine enquiry, part misjudged tease about her unstarted travels. 'Oh, I'm in Ashqabat' she says prosaically, as if this should be self-evident. I make some opaque but friendly sound to deflect attention from my geographical ignorance and misfired humour. 'That's in Turkmenistan' she explains without comebackance.

Later I look it up in an atlas: I had no idea of its existence.

*

Still later I am pondering this now ubiquitous greeting from terra firma to mobile: 'Where are you?'. Thirty years ago such an utterance was non-existent: if you called someone on the phone you also knew their location; if you did not know where they were you could not contact them. Such a question would have been nonsensical or ironic metaphor. Contact required locational, and usually personal, knowledge.

Even more has the Internet rapidly dislocated such timeless preconditions for communication. We can now convey precise and instant messages with no identifying features of person or location. The *content* is all: the *context* increasingly unnecessary or lost. As our electronically mediated messages and data become more crystal-clear, their human and vernacular ambience becomes more fog-like. This new world of combined clarity of content and obscurity of context had some early and interesting explorers. Internet sex has managed (for countless many) an astonishing uncoupling from experiences and activities mostly rooted in the primacy of the interpersonal and physically sensate. Internet users could now, with unprecedented ease, replace these with an instant, synthetic composite of the depersonalised and abstracted: a screen glowing with generic alphabetical signs (words) conveyed featurelessly (text) by an unknown person. Even the latter may be wishful thinking: such cyber-erotica could have been generated by computer. Yet even if the transmitter of virtual delights is human, that human form may have little resemblance to the one constructed by the recipient: there is no touch, sound, smell, taste, face, gaze, or even a real name. There is no evolved mutuality or history. We have, instead, highly abstracted, electronically transmitted signals, which the recipient then conjures into a desired fantasy of desire. Such are our substitutes for 'intimacy' when we choose to eliminate context with content.

Such computer-mediated dislocation inevitably darkens with opportunities for malign perversity. We are now a mere few clicks away from masking our spying, intrusions, threats and assaults on others: cyber-bullying and graphic sexually framed humiliations or terrors are the shadow of cyber-erotica.

Under a cloak of anonymity it is easy for us to do our worst: we have democratised *Jack the Ripper*.

*

Such cyber-dysrotica may be one guise of Satan in our digital age and brings to the bystanders a dark wonder of strangers, fear for our children and unsettling frissons of doubt about partners. The most egregious of these will bring us salacious headlines.

The rapid development of such social disjunctions is largely due to digital informatics. There are many other forms that are now so commonplace as to arouse little thought or comment, yet generate new types of oblivion. These oblivia usually incur losses and while the short-term effects of these may seem benign and superficial, the longer-term consequences will turn much less trivial. Here are two apparently disparate examples of evolving dislocation.

i) Where am I? Ask the Sat Nav

I am lost in a part of Norfolk unknown to me. There is a complex cluster of non-motorway road junctions with inadequate and discrepant signage that may have recently been changed and does not conform to my map. Close to the junctions is a large petrol station with several drivers filling up. I ask six drivers about the signage and designation of the nearby major roads and they are all amiably and helpfully unhelpful: they do not know.

What is happening? I think this small story is part of a new and growing trend; it would not have happened twenty years ago. Clearly, this is not yet science: my sample is small and there is no control group. I may just have been unlucky in choosing six consecutive non-locals who were all as new to the area as myself. Maybe, but I have other, similar experiences that indicate something more interesting and important is happening: just as we increasingly do not know our neighbours, we are losing personal knowledge of our neighbourhood, our terrain and location. A key to understanding this story is that most (all?) of the drivers had Sat Navs and, I believe, were decognitised by their devices. They habitually tapped in required destinations, thus delegating all navigational decisions: this leaves them 'free' when driving to wander the mind, to chat and to phone. The technology thus unburdens them: they now need little sentience of their journey and surroundings: personal knowledge of whereabouts hence ceases to have any useful function. Whatever needs to be known can be accessed instantly in the vast annals of cyberspace; omniscient and omniprescient – like a secular deity. By constructing this supra-ordinate intelligence we human users are relieved of the burdens of having to plan, notice, remember or make decisions when journeying: our surroundings become irrelevant and we are freer to go on our personally oblivious, computer-sighted way – a procession of antennaed, encapsulated cyber-solipsists.

This computer-mediated oblivion of our geography may be thought inconsequentially expedient and thus benign. I think this is mistaken: such losses may start subtly, but later the price paid is serious. This is currently becoming painfully clear when similar computer-enhanced oblivion loses sight of people.

What then happens?

ii) Who is he? Ask the computer

Stuart is sitting with me again, trembling and harrowed, in my consulting room. His partner, Jill, has brought him to the surgery with tender but tiring vigilance and now stays with us – he needs many mooring points to stop his drift out into an ocean of perils, unhorizoned and tempestuous.

Stuart is in his mid-forties and after many less catastrophic premonitory symptoms, his mental cohesion and integrity are now breaking down. He has no clear or coherent language for this disintegration: at first he described his frightening experiences in physical terms, then he learned to talk from a basic psychological but impersonal lexicon – of panics, disturbances of mood and emergency escapes by impulsive actions. Healthcarers apply their usual terminology.

Stuart's manner is of a frightened, wary, resentfully hurt child who wants to find someone to trust but fears making that decision. There are good reasons for this, which he has been encouraged to share in numbed or painful fragments. His life was conceived from a careless and doomed union by a young couple, and his father had disappeared forever several months before he was born. His young mother did not want – and then could not cope with – an infant son, but she was blessed with parents who were happy to do both these things.

Stuart had five loving, devoted, stable and happy years with these grandparents before a sudden destructive disruption: his mother found a new partner whom she wished to marry and intended to accelerate the formation of her family group by reclaiming Stuart. The loss of his grandparents was litigious and he saw little of them after the battle-dust settled. Worse was to come: his mother never conceived again and his stepfather's initial tolerance toxified through indifference to contempt and hostility, to eventual violence that ineradicably and intensely frightened and humiliated the boy. Fearful of and for her marriage, Stuart's mother colluded with the stepfather. Stuart's contiguous, through different, mistrust of men and women took root.

Stuart survived these betrayed attachments in his youth by various kinds of numbness, denial, structure and displacement – alcohol, drugs, sexual promiscuity, drunken fights, emigration, army service – but by his middle years his defences are crumbling. His estranged ex-wife and two adult sons are long lost to him and expatriated in the wake of his many years' flailing and dissonant defences; buttresses against his ancient grief, rage and mistrust. But these could bring only partial and fleeting respite – the spectres would surely return. This they did when he attempts to reciprocate Jill's wholesome and unconflicted love: Stuart's bedevilment reconflagrates, but this time he does not attempt to escape.

Instead he breaks down.

If Stuart is to now turn this breakdown into a breakthrough, he will need the kind of caring and understanding stability that he once received from his grandparents. To heal such deep and chronic wounds he will need long contact with, and containment by, a kind of extended 'loving family' in which there are several overlapping and complementary roles. For healing 'love' – a patient, non-possessive, non-controlling, benign, disinterested interest – is most fertile when it can flow between several angles and strata. Jill's love is primal, domestic and personal. What I offer is more boundaried and ritualised by professional role – though heartfelt for us both – and massively symbolically significant for Stuart: I become the benign and committed father who does not leave. But the strains on me in doing this are great: I, too, need a supportive and therapeutic extended 'family'. I will need my psychiatric colleagues to widen the net and share the strain.

But the NHS psychiatric services that I ask to help me help Stuart do not now have the kind of consciousness or organisation to step into this kind of role – one guided by powerful metaphorical realities of stable family surrogacy and loving therapeutics. Instead they offer a carouselled medley of long, formulaic interrogatory assessments, risk-management protocols, behavioural modification programmes, Treatment Plans and (transient) Care Coordinators to attempt cohesion and comprehension. These latter flail and fail: Stuart often sees someone different each time he attends, and when he does so they ask him similar and repetitive questions without, apparently, any growth of personal or mutual understanding. This is negatively reflected in Stuart's recall: he cannot remember their names, job designations or much of what was said. 'They look at the computer a lot and seem to be mainly interested in whether I'm taking my tablets and whether I intend doing something pointless or horrible. They keep on asking the same questions like some kind of Official Inspector … No, I don't think they're really interested in me, only what I might do …'

The depersonalised fragmentation of care worsens with time, as Stuart's possible attachments never develop naturally, instead they are recurrently displaced by administrative formulae, timetables and plans. Over several months he is passed between many different teams, which he cannot remember, but I do.* All of these encounters of *Therapeuticus Interruptus* add to his core sense of futile and despondent unwantedness and the inscrutable, random, uncaring, unreliability of others and their power.

Stuart understandably loses faith in them, but not (yet) in me. I make several phone calls over these months in an attempt to retrieve and repair the situation. I speak to Team Managers, Care Coordinators, Duty Desks, various types and grades of Psychiatrists and – eventually – the Clinical Director of these services. The pattern becomes familiar: the responsible practitioner may have been briefed about Stuart, but rarely know much more about him. But I am told this is not significant: 'all relevant mental healthcare workers can locate him on our shared (computer) System'. No, they cannot have a more detailed discussion with me, but my concerns will be noted for the next Team Meeting. They politely deflect my suggestion for more personal continuity of care: 'Stuart's Patient Journey is carefully considered and planned by each Multi-disciplinary Team. In all this we follow our NHS Trust protocol as an assurance. There is thus no need for any one practitioner to have the more particular knowledge or longer-term commitment or relationship you speak of. Our System will tell us what we need to know.'

Despite Stuart's lack of meaningful engagement with these professionally sequestered colleagues I still want him to attend. They may not offer what either he or I need, but at least they are around to provide a modicum, or symbolic presence, of caring: I do not want to be left to struggle as a 'single father'. Neither do I want him to collect a fresh label of 'uncooperative patient': his ancient label of 'illegitimate' is already more than he can bear.

*

I am thinking of similarities between Internet sex without personal intercourse, the Sat Nav directed drivers who can designate their destination but never know their journey, and the Mental Healthcare workers who know how to access Stuart's healthcare data but are not concerned to know Stuart. All assume a supra-ordinate system that short-circuits the need for personal connection, responsibility or sentience – all elements of *relationships*. The cyber-knowledge of the Sat Nav impoverishes our *relationship* with our traversed geography. The cyber-knowledge of the Healthcare Computer too easily replaces our *relationship* with people whose lives we accompany at critical times. The healthcarers I spoke to talked of Stuart – often, I thought, to their complete self-satisfaction – as if they had successfully Sat Naved him on his Patient Journey, and no further discussion was necessary. Such cyber-parenting may reassure the institutional healthcarers, but is experienced quite differently elsewhere. Now I must largely cope alone as a 'single father', without an extended therapeutic family. For Stuart it is far worse: his ancient history of family instability, unpredictable strangers and recurrent powerless subordinations to others' decisions is re-experienced painfully by him, but never discussed with them. Their relationship is mostly with their System; Stuart may be granted some of this, if he conforms.

*

Holism – our humanly flawed attempt to see wholes – can never be perfectable or completeable and is thus an eternally precious but doomed project. It is an aspiration, an inspiration, a philosophy and an ethos: we travel, but never finally arrive. It is the antithesis of expedience, device or procedure – although we must make compromises with these. Amidst this, holism is untidy and risky: we must employ imagination to make unobvious connections with the apparently diverse – activities that cannot be measured, managed, packaged or proved. Holism thus needs, at least, our tolerance of – at best, our creative play with – ambiguity, uncertainty and unproveability. Paradoxically, it is when we risk and venture these that we develop our most meaningful understandings of one another. Just as the Sat Nav's crisp, authoritative certainty may blind us to our geographical journey, an over-systemised, computerised healthcare system may unsight us to the hidden humanity of our fellow journeyers.

'The quest for certainty blocks the search for meaning. Uncertainty is the very condition to impel Man to unfold his powers.'

Erich Fromm, *Man for Himself* (1947)

---

*In one year Stuart was seen by the following Psychiatry and Psychology Teams: Hospital Liaison Psychiatry (three hospitals); Community Mental Health: Assessment and Brief Therapy; Mood Anxiety and Personality; Increased Access to Psychological Treatment Services; Emergency Psychiatry; Home Treatment; Hospital Inpatient; Early Discharge; Assertive Outreach.

The putative integration of fragments is called a 'Patient Journey'.

The administrative fragments themselves are propagated, defined, reified and justified by an increasing volume of tautological (often) academia, derivative algorithms, and think-tanked services-redesign documents.

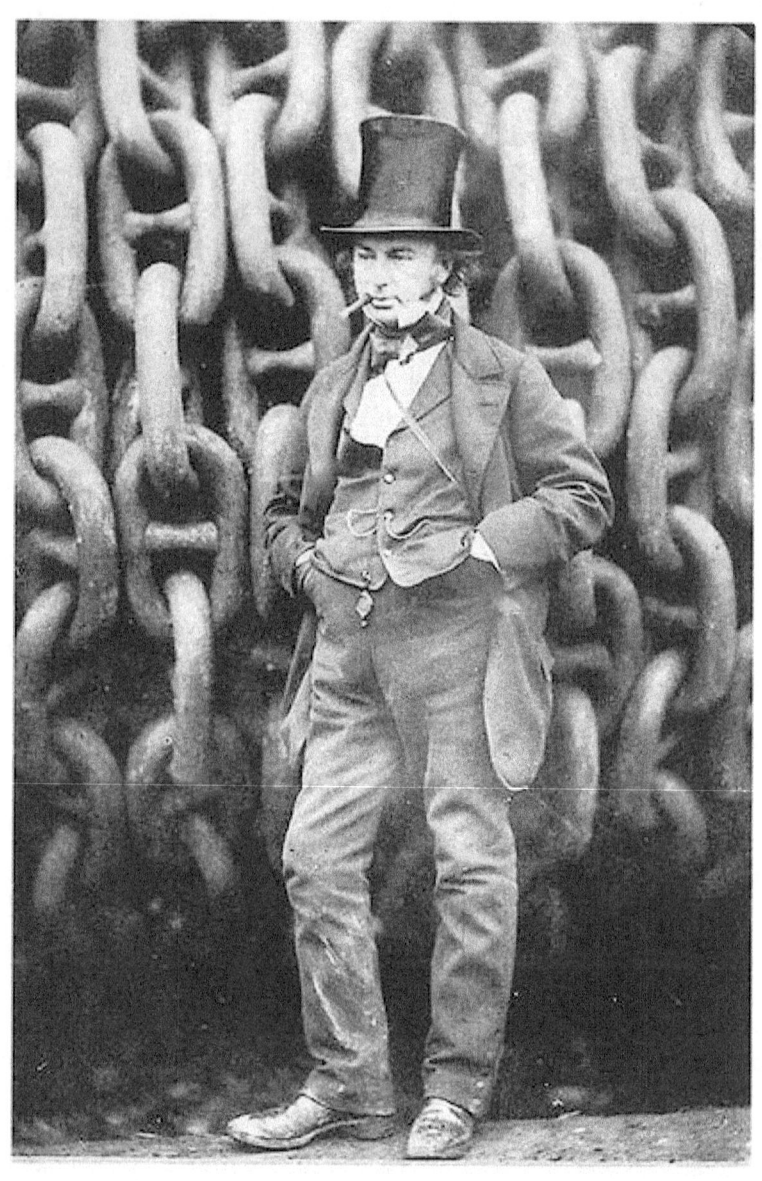

Isambard Kingdom Brunel (1806 – 59)

Edward
shot in his own interest

Technototalitarianism and
the fragility of the therapeutic dance

As long as I can remember I have been a searcher and a sceptic. This often uncomfortable predicament has led to my tendency to perspectives that are relativistic and kaleidoscopic. For a man so afflicted, my NHS practitioner roles have been contrastingly stable and durable. Nearly 30 years in the same general practice and hospital posts have offered me a remarkable long-term vantage point for the destiny of individuals, families and the tides and style of organisations and working ideologies. Through all this, my intense interest in the complexity and power of human contact and attachment has remained vital.

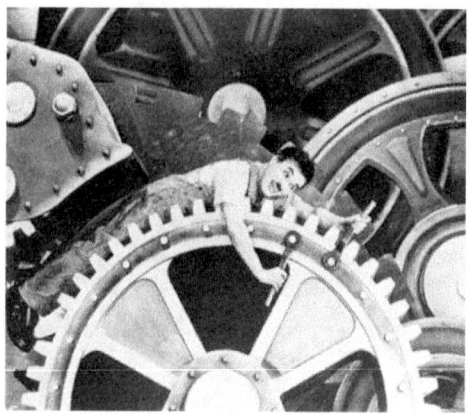

Charlie Chaplin *Modern Times* 1936

Even in slight things, the experience of the new is rarely without some stirring of foreboding.

Eric Hoffer, *The Ordeal of Change* (1964)

Change is scientific, progress is ethical; change is indubitable whereas progress is a matter of controversy.

Bertrand Russell, *Unpopular Essays* (1950)

It is well past midday. For nearly four hours I have variously survived a chimeric procession of human contacts that push and crowd a Monday morning GP surgery. I am turning light-headed, retreating with compassion-fatigue, and losing my sharper abilities for convergent thinking. When Edward enters I know I will have to recover my receding faculties, if we are both to feel well-disposed to one another.

Edward is a complex man, and has long evoked much frustrated confusion in those who attend him. His large physical frame has carried his 82 years mostly with great reliability and robustness but, I sense, without much expression or pleasure. His physical complaints of mild hip arthritis and angina have been well suppressed by usual current treatments. Not so his 'illness behaviour'. Edward's frequent attendances, over many years, despite his lack of serious illness, had first perplexed, later irritated and finally enervated his previous doctor, Dr T, a man long admired for his good-humoured restraint and diplomatic wisdom. With Edward, Dr T tired from an attrition of his higher powers; his colleagues sighed with relief when he declared an uncharacteristic abandonment of this 'heartsink patient'. They had secretly and individually feared far worse. Edward, removed from Dr T's list, was assigned to mine; a blind and involuntary coupling.

Six years later, I have identified and commiserated with Dr T, his travails and honourable self-discharge. Edward has been a 'difficult' man, often experienced as contrary and contradictory, ambiguous and ambivalent: his neediness mistrustful, his responses to attention often spiky and diminishing. Beneath this surface of confused signals and contacts, I have imagined a life of thwarted yearning, of previous struggles, and now, turbulent submission. Edward does not want his private life probed, but he does, somehow, want it understood. He recurrently declined invitations to enter the more directly investigative and interventive domains of psychiatry and counselling. Early on in our encounters I framed these suggestions, I smugly thought, with much skill and artistry. His retort was tart: *'I'm no more crazy or disturbed than you, doctor'.*

I had insight enough not to contest him. Explicit enquiry remained subtly parried. My interest in explanatory history, or explicit portraiture, would not be met. I was slow to learn that well-travelled approaches of medicine, psychiatry and psychology could not help me to help, or even contain, most of this man's complaints. I was in the world of the shaman and the cryptographer.

In the analogy of journeying, I was now confined to the use of narrow winding tracks in poor visibility over uneven, often steeply inclined, surfaces. The steady, even, well-lit, straight, broad roads of 'conventional' medical practice were elsewhere. Off the major thoroughfares, hazards are more numerous and various. To stay on such paths requires vigilant anticipation and attention. With Edward I learned to offer him not just the usual, pre-packaged questions, explanations and reassurance, but also bespoke medical ritual and respectful play. Lingering over a manual (not electronic) measurement of his pulse and blood pressure was usually unhelpful medically, but offered a form of structured, caring touch and contact that was tolerable and safe for this lonely and armoured man. 1 learned, too, of an acerbic and anarchic wit beneath his previously gruff, combative presentations: our banter developed an accompanying, unspoken affection. I was rewarded for taking The Road Less

Travelled. He agreed to come every two months for 'routine review', and stopped his more frequent opportunistic, antagonistic attendances. Receptionists reported a baffling patience and politeness. I cautiously enjoyed my brief but regular appearances in a marathon role as secular priest. Edward became less querulously hypochondriacal, his presence in the room was lighter, his gaze softer, he left the room willingly and without a trail of unfinished, unspoken business. He stopped being a heartsink patient. I thought often of the innumerable ways that we humans devise for engineering contact, but ensuring structure and optimal distance between us. Intimacy threatens more dangers than most of us wish to acknowledge.

*

When Edward enters, I am marshalling the end of my working energies. Not only must I redirect myself to our uneven, tortuous track, but I am running out of fuel. I remind myself of the probable importance of this visit for Edward, and conjure sufficient attention to satisfy us both. As Edward seats himself, there is a brief, silent peace between us. This is punctured by the imperative trilling of the telephone. Yet another distraction: I am aggravated. The practice manager's voice sounds courteously singsong but curt and peremptory: the fresh vigour of new authority, a commissar of the New Contract.

'Doctor, don't forget to weigh and measure Mr C, and put the data on the computer. You didn't do it last time, and the nurse can't do them all. I don't want us to lose points because you haven't entered the data.'

As she rings off I experience a flush of impotent, irritated resentment. Instantly, and without design, I amplify and caricature my instructions; a contagion of uncoordinated authority. I speak to Edward with unprecedented suddenness;

firmly, clipped and without compromise: 'Stand up, take your shoes off and stand over there, with your back to the wall'.

Edward, startled by abrupt change, involuntarily winces, stops his breath and jerks back in his seat, as if struck by a sharp stone. With silent obedience he stands, shoeless, where instructed in front of the measuring rule. He looks frightened and gulps.

'What are you going to do?' he asks, stiff with wariness.

'Oh', I answer with distracted new-cheeriness, 'we just want to measure you, information for the computer ... what did you think?'

Edward sags, sighs, and breathes freely with relief. 'I thought you were going to shoot me' he replies, a starkness that shocks me, before dissolving into nervous laughter that embraces us both with the recognised menace of the absurd.

Fortunately, my relationship with Edward has survived this (partly) comedic convergence of mistiming and misperceptions. I never established how much Edward's notion of his 'execution' was transient fantasy, and how much it was darkly surreal humour, mocking our relationship and my job. Aside from such idiosyncratic factors, more general and important themes can be perceived. As with many executionees, Edward was haplessly caught in a cross-current of two very different approaches, occurring at a time of rapid change and reorganisation. The first represents my efforts in the *art* of medicine: consultations that are private, individually crafted and attuned, often using data which is personal, transient and unquantifiable. This approach is at the heart of empathy, creative (more than 'satisfactory') dialogue and healing. Its language may be rich and varied, but correspondingly inexact or ambiguous. The second represented the practice manager's endeavours to impose a publicly formulated *science* to my consultation. The activity here is standardised, quantifiable, mass-produced; heedless of unprogrammed individual variables, and conveyed by language which is neutral, exact and deliberately restricted in vocabulary. Such lies at the centre of 'hard' research, treatment procedures and public health measures. Between individuals it can garner very particular knowledge, but it is unlikely, unaided, to lead to a growth of emotional or experiential understanding.

The tale has other valuable, metaphorical pointers. The practice manager's executive intrusion into, and redirection of, my multi-layered and fragile dialogue with Edward is a microcosm of many dilemmas posed to contemporary healthcare planning and provision. That systematic data-collection, measurement and 'evidence-based practice' should be a cornerstone of safe and effective practice is now axiomatic. But a cornerstone, crucial as it is to a building's integrity and stability, can only function purposefully if securely attached to walls running in different directions, which are themselves attached to other cornerstones. A cornerstone not thus related has little useful function.

Asking for Edward's height was a redundant cornerstone of activity, but one which involved team effort. At 82 years, his height can only change by amputation or involutional shrinkage. Otherwise it is a stable bit of data, of no use or interest diagnostically or therapeutically. The systems, which automatically and rhetorically demand such data, and the mind-sets and social-structures that develop in response to these, are of greater significance.

*

Sheila is the locality-manager for general practitioners in my area. More than a decade ago she had several years of various nursing experiences, and has since equipped herself for her executive role with further training in organisational management, and a wardrobe of demure, but sharp, dark suits. She is a pleasant, intelligent, open-faced woman, focused and efficient in her work. I imagine she is ambitious for promotion and will soon succeed. Currently, a large part of her job is to ensure conformity to the burgeoning requirements of the 'New Contract'. She comes to meet with my manager (Kate) and I, to 'encourage' such compliance.

Our meeting is brisk and mutually respectful, the agenda completed rapidly. This yields an unprepared and unstructured hiatus of time. I want to describe my recent story of Edward's 'execution', partly for light relief and partly because, beneath this small-scale surreal drama, larger themes and forces have aroused my curiosity and unease. The light relief comes with a gust of shared laughter.

We are laughing, I think, at the improbable and the absurd. We are laughing, also, for some respite from our own burdens, fears and spectres. The fear of harm-through-care is especially dark and universal. So, too, is the awareness of our tinsel-like autonomy, evident when we perform acts, knowing them to be futile, even harmful, because a 'higher authority' demands and monitors compliance. The example of the mandatory measurement of Edward is small but instructive. He is an intelligent, alert 82-year-old with a vigilant awareness of his bodily processes, and the kind of care he is receiving. Measuring and weighing Edward makes no sense to either him or me. It is the group's submission to the diktat of a distant planner. In themselves, these activities are neutral and unlikely to harm, but enacted in an industrialised or authoritarian manner, any procedure risks eclipsing or extinguishing more personal reflection or communication. It is hard, then, to combine mass-production with mutuality; corporate compliance with fertile dialogue.

The seismic effectiveness of applied science and mass production in the last century is matched closely by the reciprocal decline of individual craft and non-performance art. Generally, occupational activity is said to make 'progress' when individual dexterity, judgement or intuition are replaced by mechanised or electronic precision and speed. In medical practice there are areas of diagnosis and treatment where such 'progress' is hardly to be questioned: the intensive care unit, the lithotripter, the MRI scanner, are clear examples. These cumulative medical triumphs are the evolved legacy of Newton and Brunel; a medical model of applied and empirical science; biological engineering. Here 'diagnosis' is made objectively, by observation and measurement from the outside. Similarly, 'treatment' is mediated by a manipulation of 'external agents': chemicals, lasers, radiation, scalpels, stents, sutures and so on. This kind of medical model assumes engineering principles, and operates from outside the person's subjective experiences; such experiences may be dealt with courteously, but are usually thought of as distractions from the 'real work'. As with other forms of engineering, it is readily conveyed by authority, instruction, management, hierarchy, flow-charts, pie-charts and algorithms. It has its roots in scientific determinism, and has been ineluctably successful in our 'control' of many serious and demonstrable physical illnesses.

But there have always been a large (the larger?) proportion of people who seek help, but are not so afflicted. These sufferers of dis-ease, dis-equilibrium or dysfunctionality often cannot be understood or relieved by such objectively conducted bioengineering. If we are to have any success in these areas, we must somehow address the *inner* psychic and experiential world of the other; not just their fears, conflicts, fantasies and dreams, but also their positive, self-generated resources for immunity, growth and repair. Such (re)generative capacities operate at both psychological and physical levels, and are sensitive to many influences. The importance of these factors is not matched by their poor accessibility to biometric sciences. Even psychoneuroimmunology, a sophisticated sounding mouthful, often manages little more than attempts to define, in pathophysiological terms, micro-mechanisms for larger pictures, such as 'people who feel hopeless are more likely to get ill, from both trivial and serious illnesses'. It remains the *art* of attunement that helps the hopeless person feel that there can be positive possibility in contact, and to wish for a wider empowerment in their fate. It is the *art* of conveying faith, hope and charity* that can catalyse the other to heal and grow. This is a world more of induction that conduction: an inter-subjective realm of energy fields, transponders and eco-systems. Here a person's illness or difficulty may be understood and influenced by attention (not always directly) to their personal inner-world and relationships.

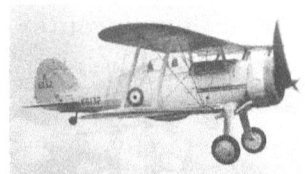

In this dimension of medical practice, the art of the consultation itself may become a powerful source of understanding and change. Like any art, it cannot always be applied, and thus cannot be mass-produced. Often it evolves by dancing in the dark; a coded bond, an improvised choreography – such activities are akin to living organisms that are delicately environment-specific. Attempts publicly to illuminate, transplant or formulate are likely, inadvertently, to distort or destroy. As in the world of agri-business, the industrialisation of living processes in medical practice can offer high yields, but there are serious dangers. We have to take care not to mutate adversely, not to poison in the process of our crop's provision and protection, not to obliterate bio-diversity in our engineering of monocultures. This latter consideration is not merely important for our aesthetics and souls; casual destruction of other life forms – 'collateral damage' – may have an amplified echo through surrounding eco-systems.

Hedgerows and trees are not just sources of beauty and wonder; they also prevent soil erosion, thus enabling our crops. Politicians, health economists and service planners necessarily make decisions for thousands or millions of individuals; their task-view is like that of the owner of an intensely-farmed vast prairie. The individual practitioner's view is much smaller, his understanding more intimate. On this scale the hedgerows can be preserved and tended; human idiosyncrasy is here both familiar mystery and essential currency.

A final squeeze on this metaphor; the practice-manager was like a 'beater', harrying creatures concealed and protected in the hedgerows out onto the open plains for dispatch. Edward's stark fantasy, 'I thought you were going to shoot me', may refer to the vulnerability of both his own life, and the few relationships that he believes sustain him.

*

My friend, Charlotte, gazes glumly to the bottom of her glass. The last drops of a mellow, fine claret. In her early 50s, she is an attractive, accomplished example of contemporary professional womanhood: bright, candid, warm, funny, compassionate, resourceful and strong. She is surprised, she says, to hear herself talk of giving up her job as a general practitioner and trainer. For years it had been a love of her life; the investment high, the rewards deep. She had not imagined changes that would so deplete her motivation, her hope.

'My last two trainees were very unrewarding. They were personable and intelligent, but really only interested in IT, devising ways of getting more data onto the computer, more 'points' for the practice ... that sort of thing. In spite of their intelligence, they have been dull in their curiosity They're not interested in the more subtle aspects of communication, the quirky humanity of our lives generally, our work in particular. At first, I thought "it's just the individual". With the second trainee, and talking to colleagues, I can see it's a trend or, worse, The Future...'

I offered her simultaneously more misery and commiseration: a sampling of my own experiences and concerns. She became encouraged by our joint gloom

'In nearly 30 years, I've never felt more deskilled. Despite my years of professional and life experience, the interest and imagination I want to bring to the work, I feel my judgement and choice are increasingly squeezed out by a kind of slavery to procedural lists and computer-templates. I feel controlled and diminished in a way that's unfamiliar for me... I now talk about my surgery as "the ants' nest...".'

*

Sheila seems a willing recipient of my lunchtime panorama. I describe the two metaphors of Edward's shooting and Charlotte's ants' nest. They usefully capture a zeitgeist, an emerging world of paradoxes where the 'ordinary citizen' is increasingly restricted and controlled by the same technology that is designed for his benefit: a high-tech cuckoo in the nest. A new totalitarianism.

Not framed by grand and dangerous ideologies, nor delivered by evil demagogues as had so shattered and terrified the earlier twentieth century, this current totalitarianism is administered by such apparently benign beings as Sheila, Kate and myself – conscientious officers in a democratic state. On reflection, all participants agree that the weighing and measuring of a healthy 82-year-old man makes no sense to any of us, but diverts us from things that do. It is the computer program that increasingly decides what we should do, and how we are performing. The individual's judgement or wish – however well-intended, designed or considered – is simply irrelevant to the computer's executive demands and monitoring. This is *technototalitarianism;* electronically coordinated mass-management.

The enthusiasts and advocates of this regime are likely to talk, realistically, of increased efficiency through compliance, clarity and precision. What they do not talk about are the unwanted side effects. At their most mild, these are manifest as superfluous and redundant activity and data; this is akin to the current over-packaging of groceries, creating waste and clutter. The more serious side-effects are those common to many command-and-control systems; they tend to run counter to flexibility and creativity. For the IT-saturated practitioner, this can easily lead to a production-lined and humanly impoverished degradation of contact skills, where individual faces are not remembered, important stories not listened to, voices not heard – the institutionalised and narrow-gazed behaviour of healthcare factory workers. Such command-and-control mindsets are inimical to the types of encounter likely to induce autonomous growth and healing. These inductions are fragile processes that require communications often more resonant than explicit, more artful than automatic.

Imaginative receptivity here is crucial and cannot be pre-programmed. In the realms of general medical practice and psychiatry in particular, consultations generated in this way lie at the heart of ancient forms of how we may best understand and help others. Many difficulties currently arise through this genus of activities being dys-compatible with mass-production, statistical research and electronic-management technologies. For all this, they require our special protection, rather than extinction through neglect and destruction of natural habitat. Treatment can be readily mass-produced; healing rarely so. Ensuring co-existence of these approaches requires much corresponding imaginative receptivity from our planners and managers.

*

It is time for us to stop. Sheila must return to debrief with her own managers; reporting on her management of me, our 'progress'. She frowns, and then purses her lips as she gathers and packs the vast scattering of data-dense papers that guided the earlier part of our meeting. She gazes at the heavy pile, symbolically I think, before turning to me, a smile intelligent with sentience and sympathy.

'You know, doctor, if you want to prosper, let alone survive, in this new era, you've just got to get on with it, like the rest of us, and not ask so many questions: you'll slow yourself down for the important work...'

This tease-in-the-tail is her offering of consoling irony, not hierarchical sarcasm. She sighs with both fatigue and, I imagine, undisclosed complicity. Her voice is less resolute now.

'I think your notions are really interesting ... I just wish we had the culture and time to really think and talk about these things.'

'Ah! Small mercies!', I mock-exalt, a small eddy of optimism, a coda: *'we glimpse democratic technototalitarianism'.*

'What?!' she says, but her frayed response is more exhausted exclamation than enquiry.

We are both, for now, too tired and busy to attempt an answer.

*

He who is being carried does not realize how far the town is.

Nigerian Proverb

Ω

---

*Faith, Hope and Charity were the names given to three obsolete Gloster Gladiator biplanes which defended Malta in June 1940 against a vastly more modern and numerous Axis bomber force. Against overwhelming odds Faith, Hope and Charity on several days harried, parried and dispersed the attackers, with great courage, skill and guile. This created a seemingly miraculous hiatus, which ensured the survival, and then recovery, of the autonomous Maltese population. The wider implications of this were fascinating and enormous. Possible healthcare analogies here are legion.

Publ. in *Journal of Holistic Healthcare* Vol.2 Issue 4 Nov. 2005

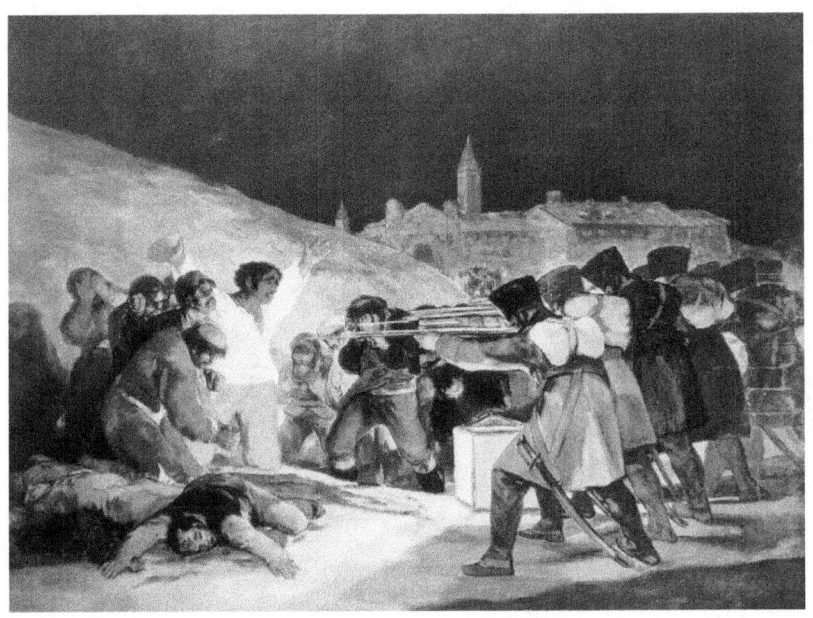

Francisco de Goya *The Third of May*, 1808

This Patient reputedly did not survive.

Planning, Reform and the Need for Live Human Sacrifices

Hegemony and Homogeny as Symbols of Progress

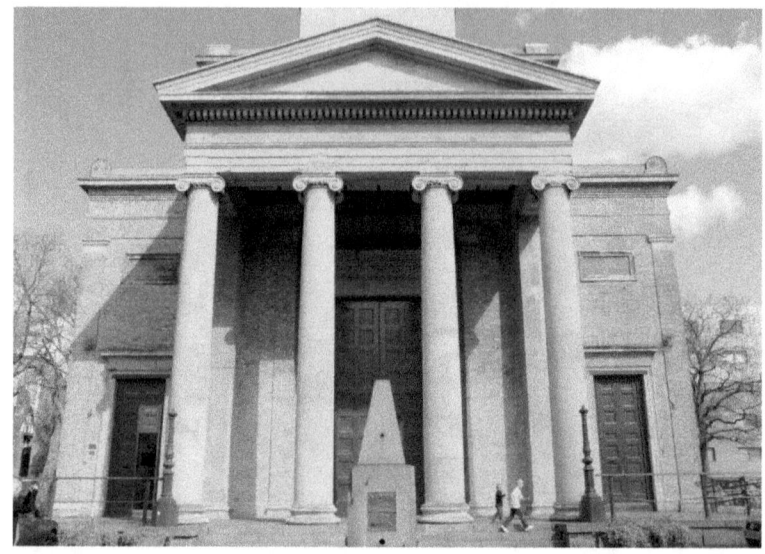

St James Church, Bermondsey, London
Home to an NHS GP surgery for nearly 30 years.

Zealous or rigid attempts to get others to standardise or 'modernise' are often shrugged off as a kind of Zombie-Curse of large organisations. But what are the hidden psychological and social currents that so burden and reduce us? How does it start? Who is responsible?

Biographical Note

I have spent most of my four decades in the NHS as a single-handed GP and part-time psychiatrist. I was always interested in the subtle shifts and balances required between opposites, to make our better understandings and interventions. Central to these is the general truth of the species ('science') *v.* the particular variation of the individual ('art'). As electronic technology makes mass management of communications and information more efficient, I fear the loss of creative diversity to increasingly standardized, anonymised procedures, professionals and premises. I fear the loss of art in medicine and heart in practice.

Prologue

Inescapably, the world becomes more populous, and our lives longer and more complex. Governments' responses tend to increase goals and targets, directives and legislation. Official policy turns easily to officious practice. There, any holistic considerations are disregarded in favour of visible submission to itemized edicts.

In healthcare this can, paradoxically, be discouraging, even destructive of best practice. Such requires conditions of flexibility, discrimination and personal investment. Institutions, by their nature, require homogeny and hegemony. Inevitable tensions arise between the institutional and the interpersonal whenever there are large-scale and complex human variables. Dextrous and imaginative care is needed to navigate and balance between these. A current narrative of an anomalous NHS practice, and a brief sampling of other, darker times, serve as metaphors to explore these themes. The descriptions, events and encounters are authentic. Usual devices disguise the characters only.

'Our sense of power is more vivid when we break a man's spirit than when we win his heart'

Eric Hoffer (1954), *The Passionate State of Mind*

'The wise become as the unwise in the enchanted chamber of Power whose lamps make every face of the same colour'

Walter Savage Landor (1824-58), *Imaginary Conversations*

When I sought sanctuary, twenty years ago, in a large, fadedly-handsome and age-weary 1830 church I was equally amused and bemused by my fate. The previous lease for my General Medical Practice had been terminated in rapid and unforeseen circumstances. Amidst my anxious and fevered searchings I found this cavernous, deserted, forlorn space. Despite the superficial decrepitude of neglect, I immediately sensed an august serenity, a rare comforting quiet in this ancient recess. As an agnostic Jew, I chuckled at my location and fortune. I was in my fortieth year.

Those early omens foretold a fertile and appreciative relationship between occupants and space. At the start of these two decades I resettled my practice and celebrated my feelings for my occupational new home with a profusion of delights for the eye and comforts for the body: impressionist and expressionist period prints, hand crafted and painted objects, plants, substantial and comfortable furniture, warm and luminous background colours. All recorded and amplified a long and loving investment: the satisfactions of the patient gardener.

This eccentric locus and mode of institutional healthcare has provoked a steady stream of spontaneous comment. Most often people would speak, with surprised warmth and bright-eyed delight, of the informal, inviting ambience, its oasis-like incongruities. Very rarely I was encountered by surly, malcontent modernism: 'What are you doing in an old building like this? Can't the NHS afford anything better? ...' These brief, cold gusts were rare, but they chilled me: I somehow knew they were harbingers of a vigorous new culture, sharply focused and uncompromisingly business-like. From the fragile peace of my oasis I glimpsed the approaching dust-clouds of new orders and reform.

*

The NHS surveyor's report felt like a thud of both inevitability and threat. Amongst the many alleged deficiencies or aberrations of 'current acceptable standards' stood an obelisk of 'lack of provision for the disabled, especially access and WC facilities.' There is no counter-balancing comment on the unusually aesthetic or comfortable environment and its great popularity among staff and patients (including the disabled), which are much in evidence. To the uninitiated, the report conveys a picture of neglect, negligence, hazard, drear of the premises and certain abject discomfort (and worse) of its occupants. This is not a place for safe or viable contemporary medical practice. This is the view of an expert on premises with a narrow, executively prescribed brief, who does not speak to its inhabitants.

*

What of the inhabitants of this alleged nest for potential mal-function: myself, my many staff, my two-thousand patients. The human eco-system of perpetrators, victims, both?

The unheeded evidence is decisively and dramatically opposed.

In summary: Results from my patient-experience questionnaires have been consistently and exceptionally good, and among the best on record. Most of my various staff (nurses, assistant doctors, receptionists, administrators etc) stay for many years, leave on good terms and have little sickness leave. I, myself, continue blessed with good health and have never taken sickness leave or had a substantial complaint made in twenty years. There has never been a significant accident. Disabled patients have cheerfully accepted help with access (when needed), and our explanations and apologies regarding any difficulties (when needed). 'It's worth it,' they have said, 'I prefer to come here …'

Holistically, this eco-system is working well in its anachronistic home.

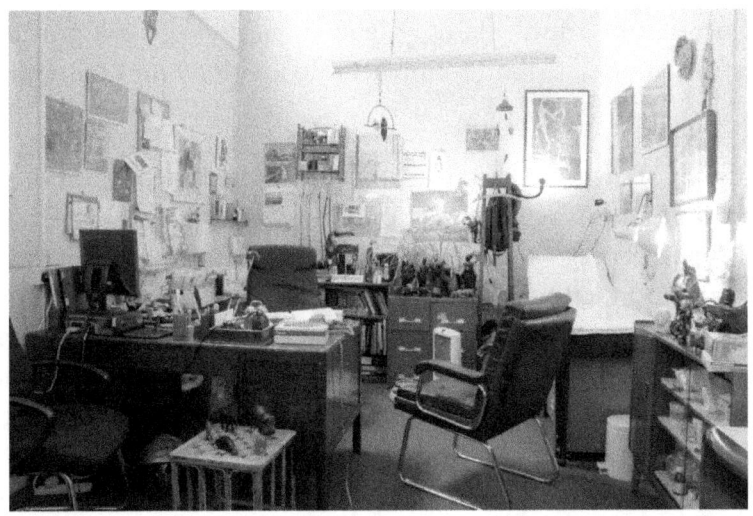

*

If 'bad' premises are defined as those likely to lead to a 'bad' effect on its occupants (surely the most meaningful definition), how can we best understand a 'bad' premises (as defined by an expert surveyor) hosting remarkably 'good' results (as defined more holistically by medical and personal feedback)? When expected correlation breaks down (as in my practice) which set of data and concepts should be discarded, and which retained and valued?

*

It occurs to me that much of this management difficulty arises from a confusion between 'correlation' (a 'sometimes' relationship, which allows exception of many kinds) and 'equation' (an 'always' relationship, often causal, that allows no exceptions). At its best such confusion may lead to clumsy, indiscriminate decision making. At its worst it is a major source of the most frightening and destructive human acts. There is a spectrum from dogmatic over-inclusiveness, to fanaticism and elimination of the most horrific kind.

Correlation mind-sets may lead to aspiration and guidance. Equation mind-sets tend to intractable ideology and mandate.

*

I do not need persuading that disabled people and their needs (among numerous groups) have been poorly understood and represented. I see clearly how improving awareness, dialogue and facilities can help them with their predicaments.

I point out to my managers that I am a relatively small inner-city practice in an area where patients have many practices to choose from. The disabled patients I have are all intelligent, informed adults who understand my predicament (lovely old building, very difficult to radically transform etc) and are well able to make their own choice. They choose to stay.

I also point out that with the cumulative growth of newer premises designed with full disabled facilities, that the problem is bound to disappear. Older practitioners and their premises will be naturally retired, to be replaced by more contemporaneous designs. With guidance and careful projected planning, the provision for the needs of this group (and others) will grow solidly and surely. There is no need for ideologically postured coercion, or destruction.

What, then, is the need for an urgent cull of the obsolescent?

*

In my frustrated dystopia I seek the counsel of two NHS managers.

The first, Sam, a genial man, stooped-before-andropause, with a passive, damply-anxious hand-shake. He listens initially, I sense, with gratuitous fascination. Soon, he shrugs, a mixture of apology and embarrassed dismissal. He looks away. 'Look,' he says, 'I probably agree with you, but that's got nothing to do with it … I don't make the rules … I'm just doing my job …' As his voice fades away, my mind involuntarily reels back some forty years to a black and white television image of a bespectacled, unremarkable looking man in a glass armoured box in a court-room. Quiet, unassuming, clerically mannered and plausibly rational. Adolf Eichmann on trial. I shock myself and shudder invisibly, grateful that my life is of this generation. I ponder how close is imaginative intuition to paranoia.

The second, Paula, shakes my hand with a dry, sure, decisive grasp. Her sympathy has a canny edge. I sense she has a well-ordered and well-filled stock of elegantly pre-packed answers. She offers me one: 'Yes, I understand, your points are very valid … Unfortunately, our hands are tied by current legislation. We cannot allow any exceptions, as we have no power or right to exercise discrimination in these matters.'

This declaration is concise, courteous and consummate: an impeccable wrapping of political correctness. I flounder with clumsy perplexity. Surely this cannot be true: ordinary policeman arbitrate about whom to confront with (say) speeding or illicit drug use. This happens thousands of times daily. And when were the laws on blasphemy last applied consistently? A lather of protest foams from my mouth.

She quietly listens to my foaming, looking down at a pen which she revolves between her fingers. A gold-plated rollerball; smooth hegemony. She then looks up at me, radiating a consoling, winsome smile; patient, experienced, forbearing. I understand I am misunderstanding something fundamental.

'Yes' she says euphoniously, 'but how is any of that going to help you? Authorities won't make that explicit. They talk only of official policy: "x is the law: offenders are liable to prosecution" ... Don't you see?'

I do, but I don't want to. My foam is difficult to swallow.

*

When Jed is addressing the media his voice has a tough, compact alacrity. Now, at his kitchen table at the end of a long Westminster political day, he sounds wearily ironic.

He had earlier been humoured though harangued by my semi-parodic analogies of contemporary politically fuelled NHS reforms with 1930's Soviet Five Year Plans. We share a fascinated scholarship of the follies, horrors and genius of the 20th Century.

'I'm a happy Kulak', I lampoon-protested. 'I'm productive and settled on my small allotment... I definitely don't want to be forced onto a Collective Farm ... I don't even want to be shot'.

Jed knows that my jesting both expresses and conceals much fear, anger, and anticipatory grief about my uncertain fate. Our shared laughter dies and the mood darkens. He rises and shuffles slowly to a favourite old armchair, a trusted friend to contain and support his strong but work-enervated frame. He well understands my relationship with the old church. He unbuttons the top of his shirt, a further loosening of the bonds and demands of public service.

'We politicians, planners and change-merchants often make almost impossible tasks even more difficult ... One of the things that happens is we lose the bigger picture, and with that much else goes; flexibility, creativity ... our imaginative humanity. But difficult change often needs a lot of effort and resolve. So, we change-merchants, and our buyers, both need evidence of 'progress', to keep going (and keep our jobs). This easily leads to the kind of deception and self-deception that, decades later, startle us with grandiose ideology and then the eventual grotesque cruelty ... The Communist Commissars developed such a strong belief in the Collectivization Programme that they would go to any lengths to ensure recruitment and conformity. The human cost, and even the clear evidence of tragically large production losses, became utterly eclipsed by the enormous ideological bulk of "The Plan" ...'

'What's often most frightening is how sincere, vocational and visionary the agents of change can believe themselves to be. People often think of Nazi SS Officers or Stalin's Communist Commissars as being sadistic opportunists. The truth is more shockingly ordinary and paradoxical: they often truly believed they were making the world a better place. 'Doing what needed to be done.' Many were sincere ideologues who needed 'evidence' of their success.'

I consider my own current drama: massively small and benign, in comparison. I think about the predicaments and modus operandae of my NHS Managers whose reputations, jobs, mortgages, maybe even self-esteem may depend upon offering up (to their managers) visible tokens and totems of change. To leave me be, in my benign and atavistic place, would be symbolic of their inertia and inactivity as agents of change. Allowing natural evolution through retirement might feel and appear like managerial impotence. A live human sacrifice will propitiate.

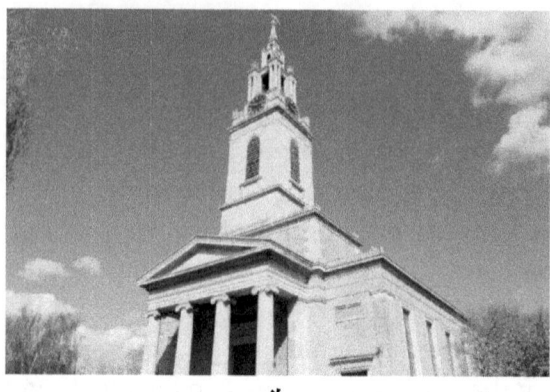

*

'How do we maintain vision, momentum, resolve *and* caution, flexibility, openness all at the same time?' A rhetorical question, Jed knows. He groans, a tiring acknowledgement of his insoluble dilemmas, the conundrae of power.

'On reflection, I don't think I'll bother any more ... I'll just sit here, where I have peace and quiet ... ', he pats the arm of his old chair, his comforter and container. He darts me a witty mischievous smile, a mock-surrender to my self-interested, insistent doubts and questions.

We sit in a restorative silence. Jed, I think, needs some respite from clamour and challenge. I want time to assimilate this bigger picture to my own small story, so important to me.

As my mind recedes from its 20th century panorama and returns to my current preoccupations, I think again of how fortunate I am to be living where and when I am.

In my fortieth year I chuckled insouciantly at my fortune. In my sixties I am less mirthful, but more mindful. The consolations of ageing are hard-won and subtle.

*

'Conformity is the ape of harmony'
Ralph Waldo Emerson (1840), Journals

Ω

Publ. *in Journal of Holistic Healthcare* Vol. 9 Issue 3 2012

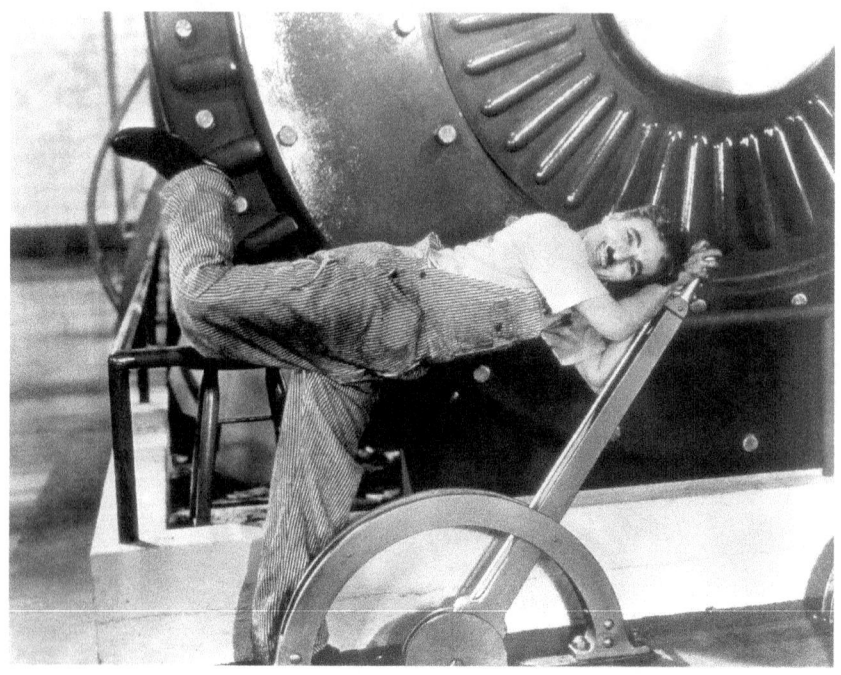

Charlie Chaplin – *Modern Times* 1936

Modern Times

(True) Parables
from the frontline of the NHS

Introduction and summary

The massive expansion of the NHS has led to a burgeoning of organisational and procedural changes deriving from mass-production industries and corporate capitalism. This 'industrialisation' of Health-Care is likely to confer clearest and greatest benefit when dealing with well-defined bodily complaints, 'physical pathology'. When dealing with the evanescence and complexity of human unhappiness or mere dis-equilibrium, 'functional pathology', considerably more difficulties are encountered and generated.

Such disorders as those of behaviour, appetite, mood or impulse ('BAMI') introduce innumerable human variables, and from all participants involved. Measurement, standardisation and technical language all become highly problematic, if not contentious. Ensuing operational difficulties are inevitable. For those interested in ethics and epistemology, important questions arise. This presents a vast and ambiguous area, particularly in General Medical Practice and Psychiatry. Inadvertent damage may result from indiscriminate and automatic use of mass-production protocols. The cost, in both human and economic terms, is probably enormous, but receives little attention.

In all human life inevitable compromises have to be made: between structure and flexibility, control and creativity, Group conformity and individual integrity. Such dilemmas have a universal span from the lives of individuals to the largest groups.

From the basis of current NHS events, these and related themes are illustrated. The narrative and dialogues are authentic. Only peripheral descriptive detail is changed to guard anonymity. Although the personal nature of the recording may be uncommon, the dilemmas they describe are not.

1. Imagination

You can't depend on your judgement
when your imagination is out of focus

Mark Twain, *Notebook* (1935)

'This one's going to be trouble ...'

Sophie approaches my desk with officious pleasure, a privileged messenger of bad news. As senior receptionist she opens and pre-digests much of my post, both to prime and protect me. Or so she supposes.

'You've been assigned this man, Stefan M, because he was extremely rude, and threatened violence against Dr K ... Dr K had no option but to remove him from his list ... Dr K's surgery had to call the police ... I hope you won't keep him longer than you have to ...'

I sense in Sophie not just concern, but a hidden, elliptical gratification, an anticipation of righteous vindication. Her expression carries gravitas skewed by a faint twist of a smile.

*

Stefan M's self-introduction to me, the next morning, disturbs me with the unexpected. His proffered handshake is warm and firm; receptive but not at all overpowering. Watching him walk across the room, I am reminded of an ageing, wounded male lion – previously a powerful predator but now incrementally vulnerable and unable to hunt. He meets my gaze with subtle and kaleidoscopic complexity: pride, hurt, defiance, pleading, enquiry. His intelligence is sharp, sprung, mobile.

The answers to my opening salvo of routine medical questions further alerts me to the breadth, depth and weight of this man's troubles. Among my notes I write:

Medical: Age 38. Heart attack last year. Lassitude and weakness since. Says he can't work because of this (never previously 'off sick'). Smokes 40/day for 15 yrs. Sister died aged 39, two years ago, amidst political asylum litigation (in Scandinavia). Psych/social: From previous African conflict zone. He and (now deceased) sister fled to different European countries as racial minority persecution mounted in danger and savagery. Both he and sister fought hard for political asylum, in different countries. He succeeded. His sister's case became impacted as a 'cause célèbre', when she died suddenly. Plight of his remaining, once-hunted family members unknown: presumed dead. Since in UK (10 yrs) worked 16 hrs/day as advocate/spokesman for his much-mauled national group. Deeply disturbed by sister's death, but worked harder and smoked more to obscure grief. Collapse of relationship with girlfriend after heart attack: says sexual potency problems (1st time) then. ?Blocked grief etc. ?Medication effect ?Smoking/vascular. Enquiries re: depression: explicitly denies this. (Tightens his jaw and hands and says: "What good would that do ... who could care for me now?" His eyes moisten, but he rapidly dabs them. He looks away – ?hoping I will, too.) Imp: ?Masked Depression ++.

I ponder this psychiatric term, now little used: an explanation, a description, a hypothesis spawning its own questions about the masker and the maskee, the relationship of the 'ghost' to the 'machine'.

Stefan M's cumulative life-traumas seem enormous, matched almost by his formidable courage, resolve and wilful integrity. Almost, but not quite. It is the 'not quite', I suspect, that has led to his incapacitation. Fighting against such mountainous adversity for so long, he has attempted an indefatigability of the superhuman. Only his body can stop him.

*

Only later, when Stefan has mapped me as a Safe-Haven, do I enquire about how his (mis)communications with Dr K had become so conflagratory.

'He told me that, from the information he had received from the cardiologist, there was no reason for me to stay off work … he asked me psychiatric-type questions, which I felt patronised by … When I tried to discuss this with him, he turned away from me toward the computer where he was consulting investigations and some kind of recommendations. I said I just can't work with this weakness I have. He said that, from the information he had, he couldn't help me further. While still looking at the computer he asked me to leave.'

I asked Stefan if Dr K had known much, or anything, of his story.

'No, he didn't ask much, and I didn't think he was the sort of person I could talk to … He seemed much more interested in what was on the computer. After he had glanced at me, I don't think he could remember what I looked like …'

*

Soon after, I attend a local medical meeting, a congregation that owes its longevity more, I suspect, to the reliably good curry served there (a silently appreciated bribe by International Pharmaceuticals), than to important shared concerns and commitments.

Dr K and I are long familiar cohorts. He is a 'busy GP' with a large practice and a bluff, no-nonsense, impatient amiability to help his long-term survival. Our affinity is stable and considerate, but not deep. In greeting he shakes my hand, a limp detached ritual as he looks away, toward the banqueted table, his gaze dully observant.

'Bad luck! I hear you've been assigned that very rude and troublesome man Stefan M, ' he mocks, with the relief of the released.

Soon after, amidst the steaming fragrances of massed curries, I try, with lightness and diplomacy, to interest Dr K in how our own common aggravations may easily blind us to the exceptional tragedy of others. He glances at me briefly with a slight twitch of a shrug, while spooning another large self-serving of Chicken Dansak:

'You like all the difficult ones,' his jest seems half-tribute, half-consolation, 'I just think some people are impossible'.

2. Belonging

Every exit is an entry somewhere else

Tom Stoppard (1967) *Rosencrantz and Guildenstern are dead*

Karen greets me by her bed, B23, with the social facility of a TV chat-show hostess. Her hair is dark, wavy and lustrous; a generous and sensuous frame to a soft, cherubic face. In counterpoint, sharply mascaraed eyes warn me of other agendas, of danger. Given the seriousness of her overdose a day previously, this now silk-gowned young woman seems disarmingly urbane and insouciantly welcoming.

Behind the curtained screen Karen and I are now invisible to the gaze and traffic of the ward. This seems to free Karen to hesitantly disclose a little-known self, more usually obscured by her competent, voluptuous masks or painful shards of self-harm.

The brief, typed referral form had forewarned me of the latter: '3rd serious overdose, with alcohol binge, in recent months. Recent stresses: break-up with boyfriend and alleged rape (different relationships). Denies mental illness and wants to leave ...'

The story Karen tells me is as perplexingly discrepant as her calm social persona and her juxtaposed, profoundly hazardous behaviour. Within the envelope of her salubrious suburban home, her publicly polished, professionally respected parents were locked in decades of a grimly hypnotic power struggle. Their two children became both weapons and casualties. Common emotional violence would erupt, often through a haze of alcohol, in periodic convulsions of physical violence. In her early teens, under cloaks of darkness and alcoholic amnesia, her father culminated the domestic damage in a sexually intrusive visit to her bedroom. Karen, with admirable but precocious resolve, left her parents and never returned.

*

This first time I meet Karen she is entering the Eye of the Storm that will determine her mortal existence. In the months that follow, her life is like a narrow path skirting the edge of an abyss. Several times she lunges, with angry despair, both softened and fuelled by alcohol, to her own self-annihilation. The serial projects of foiling her self-killing are administered by teams of physicians and psychiatrists at various other inner city hospitals: the Blue-Light Ambulance disgorges this dangerous cargo with blind haste. Precedent is neither known nor important. The practitioners immediately charged with saving her life are similarly blinded by emergency: there is no place here for nuance or finer historical reference. Medication and the Mental Health Act will contain: if not, 'Severe Borderline Personality Disorder' will explain. Karen becomes both lost and lime-lit by the doctors' (self?) defensive conferral of 'dangerous mental illness'. She may be transiently contained, but she is not understood.

This follows a pattern where the (usually) young and inexperienced practitioners, fearing for both Karen's life and their own professional career, act with zealous and crisp efficiency. In order to forestall disaster, Karen becomes crippled by pre-emptive strikes: Sectioned, medicated, monitored, 'specialed'. Karen is managed: dialogue is discarded.

Karen remembers the earlier exchanges she had with me and re-contacts my small department, a different venue and culture from the busy, bustling, prescriptive Community Mental Health Team now in charge. In this small, relatively quiet hospital department, there is great stability and accessibility for Karen. Over several years she keeps deliberate and regular contact with me via my long-serving secretary, Dorothy, a woman of unpretentious warmth and robust but respectful intelligence. Her considerable range and length of life experience may discretely illuminate, but will not dazzle. Dorothy and I are both gently silvering with age, a source of wistful banter between us.

*

The consultant in charge of the populous but constantly changing Community Mental Health Team, Dr Q, thinks more management is called for. He writes: 'We need to rationalise and unify this woman's care. It is clearly not in the interests of the patient or the Service for her care to be fragmented. For this reason, I have asked the patient to continue her attendance to this department and arrange cessation of her sessions with you...'

I telephone Dr Q in an attempt to widen our understanding of this alluringly haunted young woman. He is more interested in speaking as Commanding Officer: Karen's care would now be systematically planned, coordinated and monitored by his Multidisciplinary Team at HQ. With well-manicured authority he instructs me about the incipient New Order. Dialogue is skilfully bypassed. I am aware of holding my breath; I feel I, too, am being processed.

Karen's compliance to such prescription is fragile: she meets with the many mental health professionals assigned to her, but is progressively confused and wearied by their complex and rigid protocols, their unpredictable impermanence. She describes it later: 'They were all different, of course ... A few I thought I could really trust and talk to, but twice they suddenly disappeared – gone for another job or training, or something. It hurts and I don't feel safe ... my barriers go up again ...' Karen's offerings there turn shell-like: she yields only what she must.

She seeks connection and asylum where she feels less diminished and defined: she is discretely resolute in her regular contact with myself, and thus Dorothy. I have some unease about colluding with her unusual dissent. Dorothy and I are now as Foster Parents to this grown woman, with the added illicitness of an extra-marital affair. I convolute my mind with a cabal of dark interpretations: Freudian Triangles, Deposed Fathers, vengefully reprised children. I do not exonerate myself from these constructions: I can locate enough of my residual developmental sediment to secure my place. I have training and imagination enough to ascribe a variety of such roles to each of us. It is all plausible. It is, professionally, the safest thing to do.

I take the riskier course: I follow Karen's thoughtful dissent, sensing that she has an instinct now to create new and positive patterns. I remember a harsh and pithy judgement of a non-medical friend: 'The problem with most psychiatry is that, at best, it can stop some "bad" things happening … but it doesn't usually help people heal and grow …'. I had ruefully agreed, hoping I might be an exception, at least sometimes.

*

The months that follow bring a seemingly impossible mix of alarming headlines and growing peace. The first headlines shock with a precipitous, ill-judged but highly-charged affair. She embarks on this with an impecunious, unrooted, political Balkan refugee. Unwary, he enters a Lioness's Den of erotic attachment. With dismayed foreboding, I see her demeanour transform from a soft mist of adoration and total trust, to a terrifying furnace of raging accusation, incandescent disillusion, Total War. I see him briefly at this time: he is emotionally stunned, lost and inchoate – signs of Emotional Blast Concussion.

Amidst these emotional explosions she announces her pregnancy, her first. This news invokes waves of alarmed consternation across professional networks. How will this demonstrably unstable woman deal with the inexorable changes and responsibilities? Professional anxiety and vigilance increases. 'Risk-Management' becomes the gravitational nucleus round which their many activities orbit.

*

Karen then confounds and disarms us with her peace: a rapid crystallisation of structure and stability in her life. Faster than we are able to comprehend, she ceases her many ways of imperilling, alarming or punishing herself. Increasingly her emotional intelligence turns from hurt wariness to a capacity for reflective receptivity.

'I'm a mother now ... I have to make sure I don't pass on my mess to the next generation,' she says, patting a ripely-pregnant belly. The sagacity here is fresh and self-realised: the integrity of such self-regeneration rapidly renders obsolete the hundreds of pages of specialist, 'expert' communications in her thick folder. In this forest of technically-dense, bureaucratically-moulded prose, it is difficult to discern much of this woman's unique bondage, suffering, struggle and quest for suffrage in her own life. Seeing her now tenderly touching her belly, and uttering such protective and far-foresighted intentions toward her 'accidentally' conceived foetus, I am suddenly and rapidly connected to her in my understanding.

*

Two years later I am talking with Karen of ordinary but crucial problems: of the difficulty of being a single mother, of being receptive to her toddler-son when fatigued and already multitasking, of finding a pragmatic, appreciative semi-detachment from her son's father, her ex-lover. I have been close to formative events; she is relieved by the common understanding we create without lengthy explanation. Since motherhood, her female demeanour has changed from alluring siren to fecund and earthed mother. Sean, her delightful wide and sparkle-eyed son babbles happily in playful exchange with Dorothy, who welcomes this heart-warming, brief transformation of her office into a crèche.

Karen tells me of growing good contacts she has with other professionals: a Health Visitor, the new Clinical Psychologist, a Community Support Worker. She talks of them with growing trust and faith. Without deliberate design she has assembled around herself a kind of extended family. I reflect on this a while, and lightly contrast her flowering conviviality with our previous shared era, a tangled and dangerous time, when any dependent relationship was likely to carry an explosive charge. For several years, she had managed, time and again, but without any conscious intent, to replay myriad variations of her painful childhood dramas. As we sample these shared historical events, we contrast our different recollections and perspective. We talk of the inevitability of personal relativity, and the importance of creating common language, the most reliable balm for humankind's painful awareness of our individual separateness and mortality.

Equally surprising, to Karen and myself, is the redemption and resumption of her parents' relationship, both with Karen and one another. After many painful years without contact, her mother and father are back in her life, but dramatically transformed. They visit and welcome as calm, kindly, ageing parents and doting grandparents. Karen learns of the paradoxes behind the transformation: her parents are living separately, but close. After decades of internecine marital strife, they have found affectionate and loving peace in separation.

I marvel at the mystery of unseen and insensible matrices that guide such parallel events.

*

'A good 'Clinical Outcome', then?' Keith gently teases me with mock managerial formality and falsely dry tone. Another veteran practitioner, he, too, struggles to maintain his élan vital amidst the increasing constriction of institutional rules, diktats and deadlines; the rhetorical boa of planners and politicians.

'Seriously, though, what do you think most helped Karen's transformation?'

*

I ask Karen.

She looks down for a few seconds. I imagine she is rapidly respooling the last five years. Her answer is scattered, but thoughtful:

'You gave me time and space, faith and guidance ...' She hesitates, checking for my understanding. I believe I do, but I prompt her elaboration.

'Well, you've always been here for me, and for a very long time ... You helped me find my voice and rediscover a self I'd been running away from ... If you ever offered me guidance or suggestions, I've always thought it's from a real and growing knowledge of me, not some theory, or book or plan about The Mentally Ill ... I'm not mentally ill, I was very disturbed: it's very different...'

This notion is expressed with a brief burn of sardonic anger. This yields to a smile of recognition between us. I raise an eyebrow; my curiosity about her distinction.

'What I mean is ... Yes, I was like a person blinded with fear and confusion, and like a dumb person in not being able to talk about it. But I was never deaf: through talking with me, you guided me back to my voice and my vision. Then I could get my life back and start to make it really my own. Can a seriously mentally ill person do that?'

Her question is genuine. I delight in her simultaneous ingenuousness and sophistication. I wish often that my colleagues would ask such trenchant but unaffected questions. I inhibit my urge to now explore this question, a favourite haunt of mine. She goes on, to talk of Dorothy and our small department.

'Dorothy has been great ... always helpful and interested, but never bossy. A lot of the psychiatrists have wanted to control me, without understanding very much at all. Some have talked to me as if they know everything already. I felt very diminished: "shrunk to fit" their professional theories and procedures.

'Coming up these stairs to be greeted by Dorothy's friendly manner, sitting in this cared-for space, surrounded by growing plants and homely, colourful prints, has somehow given me the same kind of messages that I've talked about with you: that I can heal and grow ...'

She becomes quietly thoughtful, and I enquire about why she thought she had received these vital messages so rarely.

'Well, a lot of doctors don't seem to think like that, but even if they do I've got to have a good relationship with them for it to mean anything ... It's like talking about love.'

This last utterance was a short circuit I had not expected. The shock enlivens and awakens me. In unmanaged and unengineered contact, human electricity can flow in unexpected ways.

*

Keith talks of the death of a neighbour. She had lived many years in the large multi-occupancy house next door. He has only just heard of her death, three months after the event. He is disturbed by his remoteness from someone so close. We discuss the broader theme of how new technologies lead us to live such lives: where we communicate electronically-mediated words and images instantaneously to the other side of the world, but are insentient of our surrounding environment, oblivious of our neighbours.

My mind returns to an event Karen described three years ago, shortly after one of her turbulent stays in Dr Q's unit. She had resisted a brain imaging scan, feeling both repelled and afraid of the formidable machinery. The young doctor, she said, was curt, prescriptive and didactic: it was 'imperative to exclude significant pathology' (such was most unlikely, and thus hardly 'imperative'). Karen submitted to the scan, but never trusted them with much of her story.

This brief tale can be readily dismissed by more common or cursory analyses: the doctor was inexperienced, busy, unimaginative; or Karen is oppositional, oversensitive, paranoid. Much more interesting is this account as a microcosm, cultural metaphor, Zeitgeist. We are constructing a world of sharp new paradoxes and polarities. We have grown used to, expect, rapid and precise information and images: we are impatient and intolerant of the indistinct, the ambiguous, the slow. We pour massive resources into machinery to provide us with such unprecendently detailed and accurate images, but hardly notice that our own subjective image-making, our imagination, is atrophying. Karen is more easily electromagnetically scanned than imaginatively heard. Keith e-mails unknown people with effortless regularity across continents, unaware of his long-term neighbour's slow death, fifteen yards away. We increasingly delegate our tasks and responsibilities to inventions which save us time and effort but, with cruel inversity, we observe our lives as incrementally more rushed and less savoured. The mostly inexplicable, but thriving, new syndrome of children with Hyperactivity/Attention Deficit Disorder may serve as a pathological index of our accelerating, kinetic and rootless lives. To belong, we have also to be-long; we have to stay, be still and receptive.

Long enough to relate and to bond.

Ω

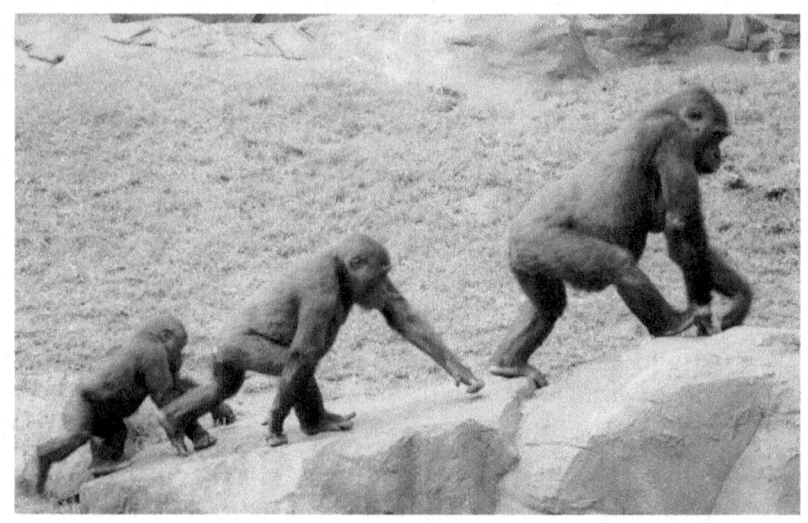

No Country for Old Men

The Rise of Managerialism and the New Cultural Vacuum

'Knowledge is proud that he has learned so much; Wisdom is humble that he knows no more.'

William Cowper, *The Task* (1785)

My early apprenticeship in psychiatry, from the early 1970s, was blessed and guided by two older men, my supervising consultants. These fatherly mentors were models for compassionate and creative professional dialogue: head, heart and soul interwoven seamlessly into their many-faceted communications. Although young and otherwise restless, I valued the cultures and communities they 'fathered' and wished to prolong their influence on me. Between them, I stayed five years. Now, more than thirty years later, I evoke these mentors and memories with warmth, admiration and gratitude: sweet–sad clouds that guide me still.

Dr G was a South African Jewish man whose family had fled Nazi Germany. As a young adult he became increasingly troubled by his comfortably privileged status in the Apartheid State. The two types of authoritarianism confronted him with resemblances, if not equivalence. To live more amicably with his conscience, he shipped his young, burgeoning career and family to England: he would train as a psychiatrist here, in the Mother of Democracies.

Fifteen years later I joined him, to begin my own training. This apprenticeship was in a large, grandiose late-victorian asylum, more recently poor and provincial mental hospital. He had a soft green-eyed gaze; observant, enquiring, encompassing. A sharp intelligence was swathed in a softly reticent, self-deprecating courtesy and deft, gentle irony. The beginnings of a stooped posture reminded me of his many stoically carried burdens and his ancestral losses. On many occasions we sat together to make some kind of 'assessment' of an individual's bruised and faltering struggle with, and against, their biological predicates and their existential tasks. He would listen with empathic detachment; his attention sometimes free-floating, sometimes sharply converged. Drawing together our ensuing discussion he would often say: 'I suppose we could call that ...'. His cautiously and ambivalently hued language was no accident: he well understood the inadequacy of our tools of language or science, in their assigned tasks of defining or changing complex human predicaments. When the psychiatric language seemed to offer some pragmatic guidance or clarity, he was transiently and conditionally grateful. We would talk of how easily an over-extension of our quasi-medical vocabulary would turn help into hegemony; compassionate containment into prescriptive control. We considered the seductive dangers of aggrandising our partial metaphors into didactic conclusions. I remember an especially fruitful dialogue, over coffee, exploring how the 'Lord of Language' becomes 'The Definer'. I thrived in the inviting and reflective space he created to initiate such discussion. In my youth and optimism, I did not anticipate how rare such sanctuaries would become.

*

The next mentor I sought out worked in the very different setting of a large, (then) prestigious teaching hospital. Dr R had, I thought, similar qualities to Dr G, but in a High-Anglican form. Spawned from an old and respected 'medical family' in the Home Counties, his salubrious, educated background progressed with a kind of blessed and urbane inevitability, through Oxbridge to his medical training. World War II interrupted such euphony with discords of terrible violence. As a young army doctor he tended the battle-shattered and trauma-deranged in North Africa. Earlier, at a distance, he had inferred the Black-Hole of human destructiveness, growing up in the legacy of the previous war. Now he witnessed it directly. Thirty years later he talked to me of this awakening: how a tidal wave of experiences impressed on him, as no theory could, the complex, fragile interconnectedness of all: mind and body, friend and foe, libido and mortido. Garnering whatever could help men restore and heal, he began his life-task and scholarship; to offer a sensitive but pragmatic service of 'Psychological Medicine'.

By the time I joined him, his department embodied the sophisticated pluralism of his experiences and intent. Although a busy service, covering a large General Hospital, there developed through and around such tasks an informal University of ideas. Alongside psychiatrists, I was engaged and guided by open-minded psychoanalysts and refreshingly rethinking medical anthropologists. Fertile experimentation enlisted other groups: GPs exploring the unexplicit psychological subtext of their work, medical students taking on patients for psychodynamic psychotherapy (the results were remarkably good, and probably not just for the patients). Without any higher edict, plan or mandate, we were all studying the Psychology of Affliction. Remembered now, from a current perspective, it seems almost impossible that this fecund community of learning and healing blossomed independently of any centrally directed NHS management or plan.

Dr R was tall and imposing, though he chose not to impose. His considerable intelligence and knowledge were quietly flanked by a kindly wisdom. I remember us listening to a many-chaptered, harrowing account of a woman's long and complex difficulties; how the medical and psychiatric organisations and mind-sets had habitually missed the personal meaning of her struggle. He looked up from the voluminous case-notes, weighing heavily on his lap. His blue eyes glinted both gentle humour and sorrowful recognition. 'It may be the best this kind of psychiatry can do', he had said. This was no condescending judgement, rather a stoic lament for how our complexity so often eludes our determined attempts to encage and understand ourselves.

*

In that decade, rapid technological advance proceeded amidst swirling philosophical challenge. From the structured, scholarly enquiries of Medical Anthropology and Sociology, to the more poetic and maverick challenges of Szasz, Laing and Illich, the stolidly revered worlds of medicine and psychiatry were being deconstructed. Fundamental questions regarding the relationship of subjective to objective knowledge, and of these to language, power and agency – all of these became matters for public and professional debate. As in all genuine philosophy, it was the process of enquiry and dialogue that was enriching, not the (impossible) end of providing definitive answers. I did not, then, appreciate how robustly dialogic those times were. Remarkably, I cannot remember talking with Dr G or Dr R much, or even, explicitly, about the challenging scholars or the rebellious luminaries, but they had somehow distilled their spirit for private consumption. These 'Two Wise Men' had developed a kind of potent humility, a demonstration of how wholesome (self) doubt could be harnessed to great therapeutic leverage. Philosophical curiosity need not be the reserved preserve of the leisured, or the academic.

*

More than three decades have passed. I am now older than either Dr G or Dr R when I apprenticed for them. My work in Medical and Psychiatric Practice is as near the end now, as it was in its beginnings, then. Despite, and because of, the passage of so many years and so many different experiences and influences, I value their values and modae operandae even more. But though my faith is solid, my optimism is not.

*

'Manage or be managed!' an executive young NHS consultant, Dr T, had exclaimed sharply to me in recent years when I lamented the loss of familiar forms of colleagial and cooperative dialogue. I was not sure if her remark was meant with any humour or irony, but I reflected later on how pithily it captured our changing world. Simultaneously it conveyed description, prescription, prophecy and ethos. This utterance came from a world far from my early influences of the Hippocratic Oath, or the gentle sagacious guidance of any Dr G or Dr R, or the better kinds of confederate socialism that had nourished and encouraged the NHS in its earlier years. This now is a world of corporate industrialism, large competing organisations, and the then inevitable hustling, hassling, spinning styles of authoritarian management.

*

More recently still, for the first time in many years, I am involved in disputed negotiation with, and between, mistrustfully aligned NHS Trusts. The problematic area is one which used to be called 'Psychosomatic Medicine': substantial chronic physical disease, fuelled and exacerbated by the sufferer's ongoing life-problems and conflicts. Such an association has to be discerned, not only by the experienced and imaginative practitioner, but increasingly by the (self) afflicted patient. It is an operational arena of interfaces, often paradoxical: Psyche–Soma, Subjective–Objective, Art–Science, Determinism–Choice, Procedure–Innovation, Individual consciousness–Generic biology. Unlike procedurally-based areas of medical practice, it relies on 'induction' quite as much as 'instruction', to help in the restoration and growth of resilience and health. *Induction* is the evocation and development of internal, personal resources; *Instruction* is the application of external, impersonal resources and notions. Generally then, induction is dialogic; instruction is didactic. Induction is (more) receptive; instruction propulsive. Applied with functional synchrony, they are two essential components of holistic care: like the pulsing heat; receptive in diastole, propulsive in systole.

Problems arise. The 'systolic', instructive, propulsive aspects of medical practice can be (relatively) easily measured, managed and standardised. The 'diastolic', inductive, receptive components cannot. Politicians, health-economists and planners, managers and clinical directors are likely to see the way to greater effectiveness and economy through increasing standardisation, mass-production, instructive management. The burgeoning plethora of audits, goals, targets, 'treatment packages', NICE guidelines, league tables, QUOF points – all are designed to supercharge the 'systole' of propelled, executively-managed care.

What then happens to the 'diastolic' functions of care? Diastole needs time and space for the heart to fill, for systolic thrust to be possible. Likewise, we need the time and space for the art of induction, the inter-subjective dance that makes the objective then possible. As with families, we need freedom-within-structure in order to function well, both individually and collectively.

The structure we can engineer, mass-produce, manage. The freedom we cannot. We must instead assure a respectful space, a skilled conservationism.

*

I attend this meeting of managers because my long-running 'Psychosomatic' service has been terminated by two mistrustfully allied executive NHS Trusts. This happened by oblivious default, without consultation with those most affected: the patients, referring clinicians or myself. Protests from all were parried by the kinds of skills, 'correct' avoidance and ellipse that large organisations use so frequently as a first line of defence. The new trusts, and their employees, are now part of a corporate quasi-industrial world. This confers a new, but continuing, Darwinian struggle for survival of the fittest, with all the evolutionary feints, deceptions and traps – the behaviours of threat and fear. There necessarily follow changes to our mental life; our priorities, then our values: our individual thought-process, then our collective culture.

The psychosomatic work I do may have been valued by patients and clinicians for many years, but it has not been executively planned and is thus not a contractual obligation of any trust. Occupying a territory of interfaces, it does not feature in the thrall of official goals or targets, or the threat of complaints or litigation. For the survival of the trusts, it confers no evolutionary advantage. Ipso facto, there is no problem and no need.

*

As I listen to the guarded forays, assertions and retorts of these corporate managers and managing clinicians, I am struck by their acquired sureness of style and resolve of language. In this new world of competitive commissioning, expressions of doubt, ambiguity or respectful hesitation are likely to be seen as hazardous indecision, implied submission. To survive, an aura of potency, resolve and business must be maintained. These Commissioning Officers, who are now paid to commodify and trade in areas of outstanding natural complexity (human suffering), become powerfully and subtly changed by this new kind of market economy. Trusts' negotiations and spokespersons must now appear, like senior politicians or multinational corporate bosses; authoritative, confident, decisive. The product marketed must appear definite, clear and assured. 'Confidence', as with the banks, becomes less an internal state of real assets, more of a hypnotic strategy, illusion, even deceit.

The economy determines the language.

'Providers' now spawn 'treatment packages'. Fascinatingly kaleidoscopic forms of difficulty and distress are speedily designated to 'mental illnesses' or 'disorders', and hence streamed to the 'appropriate intervention'. There is no language (or time) here for the ambiguous, the nascent, the naturally evolving; the semiotics of symptoms, the creative possibilities of uncertainty. The language is systolic.

*

And then the language determines the thinking.

The monoculture language, intended to expedite the functions of system and symptom management, does not merely provide utilitarian thoroughfare. Like tarmac roads, such prevailing or exclusive language destroys other forms of intellectual life or thought. An unmitigated use of psychiatric or organisational language will, for example, lead to reification; an unwittingly obstructive consequence of language. Mental illness becomes a 'thing', akin to a Cataract or Inguinal Hernia. Sometimes this is unrivalled in effectiveness as a guiding metaphor, a procedural template. At other times, other kinds of language and understanding will yield more: the symptom as lever, language, sacrifice, catalyst or code; the sufferer as messenger or conduit; 'illness' as encoded social or personal construct or contract. The development, and discriminating use, of a wide repertoire of such 'modae cognitiae', constitutes the bedrock of any 'Art' we may bring to our medicine or psychiatry. The heart of this art must have diastole and systole in constantly changing, but functional synchrony. When this does not occur, the interpersonal or clinical disturbance represents a kind of dysrythmia.

*

And then the thinking determines the (inter) action.

'There's only one way to manage this kind of psychotic patient...' avers Dr T in a way that seemed to impute to any attempt at discussion, qualities of incompetence, ignorance or insolence. In fact, both the patient and situation were rich with possibilities of understanding and encounter. The man's psychotic difficulties turned out to be a minor part of what responded to a more holistic and personal approach. But Dr T's utterance reflects far more than her particular nature, or her response to this scenario. It exemplifies the problems of excessive government, management and executive control in matters that are also personal, protean and delicate. The highly structured, proactive 'bullish' vocabulary and style is endemic amongst corporate captains. It now risks becoming epidemic in areas of complex human care, where it can do real harm.

*

In my many youthful years of apprenticeship to Dr G and Dr R, I never heard such sharply prescriptive or didactically summary communications. These recollections are not only about departed individuals, their sterling and subtle qualities and my long-enduring admiration. They are also about changed times and cultures, and about the loss of values that could flourish in organisations that were more collaborative, colleagial and cooperative; when doctors were more vocational and less careerist; when managers did more to facilitate and less to control.

How would Dr G and Dr R have fared in this current world, to which Dr T is so much better adapted? To my consternation, my imagination deserts me.

*

'A wise man hears one word, and understands two'.

Yiddish proverb

Ω

Publ. by *Public Policy Research* 16:2 2009

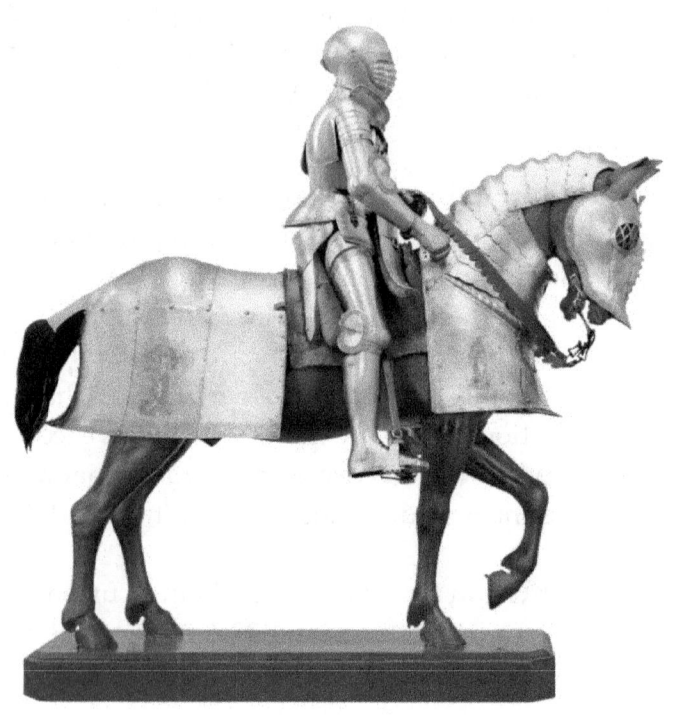

Armoured knight early 14th Century
NHS mental healthcare manager early 21rst Century?

Psychiatry
Love's Labour's Lost

The pursuit of The Plan
and the eclipse of the personal

Attempts to gain greater safety and efficiency in
Psychiatric services have led to a redesign which mimics
the increasing streaming and fragmentation of Medical
Services. The results are, very often, dislocating,
depersonalising and demotivating for both staff and
patients alike. Human and economic costs are
considerable. This article explores by narrative and
analysis.

Introduction

It is a little over thirty years since I gave up my full-time job in Psychiatry. I reduced this work to part-time, became a single-handed Principal General Practitioner and ran a small, private psychotherapy practice. Amidst this busy multivalent work, I turned oblivious and vague from the confusing mosaic of organisational plots and plans gathering around me.

The metamorphosis within the NHS would be much different to what I had indifferently supposed. More recently I have awoken to the nature and consequences of changes that incubated and hatched in this last decade, my period of circumspection.

The psychiatric service now settling is a much more complex compound of numerous, specialised, boundaried teams. These mostly operate with strict intake criteria and sharply delineated, short-term goals. Algorithmically, such a managed medley may look elegantly precise and machine-like. Such is the likely and wishful perception of managers, policymakers and (increasingly) practitioners.

This sharply contrasts with the experiences I hear elsewhere. Frequently I receive patients bewildered and adrift. They attempt to describe a plethora of different teams and formulaic, interrogatory styles of interview. I strive to counter their fatigue and dispiritedness. These often ensue from the recurrent breaking of short-term therapeutic bonds. The engineered neatness of diagnoses and clinical plans does not often correspond to the natural untidiness and inconsistencies of people's lives and distress. Or their complex and changing needs for reparative contact. Older practitioners, too, talk of their frustration; of being deskilled and disempowered in their fragile endeavours to respond with care that is personally attuned, and with an open view to the longer-term. It is not just patients who may be 'shrunk-to-fit'. These tribulations derive, paradoxically, from designs and styles of management attempting to address 'efficiency' - a Higher Good, a necessary Utilitarianism.

This collage of recollections and notions, from both General Practice and Psychiatry, serves both to illustrate and explain some major, current healthcare conundrae. The Law of Unintended Consequences is evidenced from diverse viewpoints.

Increasing hegemony and rigidity within and between institutions, at the expense of interpersonal attention and sensitivity, is a central and recurring theme. Inevitable, though inadvertent, losses to our understanding of individuals, and thus our therapeutic effectiveness, are difficult to measure directly. Indirect evidence is plentiful. It signals exponential losses to the kinds of therapeutic benefits that need quality and continuity of human contact as a bedrock. The new services are thus very much more expensive,[1] but, in crucial ways, less effective.

In the following accounts, events and dialogue are authentic. Usual devices of disguise protect anonymity.

*

I would rather ride on an ass that carries me,
  than a horse that throws me.

George Herbert, *Jacula Prudendum*, 1651

The telephonised voice is unfamiliar. It is bright, young and crisp, with the assurance and pre-set utterances of a corporate officer, officially and well briefed. Amanda tells me she is the Duty Manager for the Community Mental Health Team:

"We have had our Referrals Meeting. We have considered your letter and do not think that your patient, Tessa, meets our intake criteria. We noted that her attendance here previously was poor, and we didn't think she benefited from our Service …"

*

Three weeks earlier Tessa comes to see me, her GP of twenty years. Now in her late 30s, Tessa enters with a reticent demeanour of bruised trust and flickering hope. I have long known these to lap a larger internal land-mass of bleak fatalism and despair. She offers me a very brief direct look and a hint of a smile of greeting: I imagine she cannot risk more.

More than a decade ago I attended the multiple and fresh wounds in, and from, Tessa's family. The fewer were stark and shocking: a young brother's violent suicide, in prison; an older brother's serious residual brain damage, from drugs. Tessa, thereafter, was his Carer. The many were more 'ordinary', but cumulatively destructive: chaotic and emotionally illiterate parents, compounding their (family's) problems with alcoholic oblivion. Then the consequent physical damage. Then came disability and, ineluctably, their dependence on Tessa. As a droning bass-note: the symptoms and trap of endless, ugly, economic poverty.

Knowing something of this background and story I understand the meaningful evolution of her psychiatric Stem Cells: her swamp-like poor self-esteem, insecure attachments and default position of helpless depression. Simultaneously, I have long admired the battered and malnourished hulk of her will to survive and connect. These are the germinators of her health: I encourage them in myriad ways. Over many years I have offered her, piecemeal and compressed, refuge, reflection, and asylum. Often we have needed expedient, intermittent bolstering from others, from Psychiatrists, Social Services, Day Centres and Counsellors. Like the Asthma and Diabetes she has 'inherited', her Mental Distress is not decisively curable, though it (she) is responsive, ameliorable and containable. Mostly I guide and I palliate. Often, I help her perceive and act in ways that do not make difficult situations worse. I may sometimes help her succeed. Far too late to make major reversals of Fate, I offer valued morsels of parenting that were tragically lacking in her biological family: safety and reliability. Then space and sensitivity, for respectful, imaginative dialogue; sometimes, even, wisps of play. All have been necessary, but rarely sufficient. To alleviate some of the insufficiency, I welcomed synergy from like-minded colleagues.

*

One such was Dr M, a senior psychiatrist at the local (teaching) hospital. A little short of twenty years ago I am meeting Dr M every few months. Our conversations generate mutual interest, guidance and clarification. We share care for many puzzling, distressing or enervating patients. Our roles, locations and periods of contact are different, sometimes disparate. It is the exchange of these that may enlighten work that is so often uncertain and uncompleteable. Sometimes it will not: then there is support and affiliation from a trusted colleague; a humble balm for long-term professional goodwill and morale.

The cordiality and informality of our meetings is framed by a light lunch or early evening meal. There are no recorded agendae, bullet-points, power-points, or action-plans. This is learning by mutual enquiry; Education at its most feral and refined.

Over many years I had several such alliances with Senior Psychiatrists from this hospital. Although the style varied with the individual, the pattern of commonality endured: we were fortified by a pragmatic rapport of uncertainties. Such extemporised dialogue made us a little more able to perceive and address the chimeric complexity of people's lives.

*

I remember a conversation with Dr M about Tessa, early one summer evening. As usual, we each brought our samplings of newly garnered notions and reports. Again, his perceptive compassion and imagination freshened my own efforts, sometimes lost and stumbling. Thus enriched through our fallibilities, we grew an implicit bond of gentle, ironic affection.

Tessa, too, benefited from this unplanned but now deliberate and fertile overlap of 'multi-agency care'. I thought of the secure and happy child who senses good contact and connection between her parents, but does not necessarily know (or care) what they are talking about. Tessa partially articulated this, shortly after her brother killed himself:

"Mum and Dad can't offer one another, or me, or anyone any comfort … Thank goodness you and Dr M talk together and are here…"

Later that evening Dr M told me of mooted plans to reorganise Psychiatric Services. He was not directly involved, but had heard:

"They [the planners/authorities] think that the hospital-based services are too large, impersonal and distant (both geographically and psychologically) from the populations they serve – the frightening, forbidding 'Castle on the Hill', above us and surrounded by mist, that sort of thing.

"Their idea is to have smaller, but more community-based, centres instead. These will be 'friendlier'; they will certainly be geographically closer to most patients. Also, they will be excellently placed to build up personal working relationships with GPs and their Counsellors, Health Visitors, Social Workers, District Nurses … even Work-placement Officers and FE Colleges … What do you think?"

It all sounded good to me. My hesitations were trivial, brief and personal: I rather liked the system as it was, and my relationships within it. Also, I'd never really been interested in that kind of Grand Planning … I soon stopped my timorous muttering. I assured him I would look forward, with alacrity.

*

Twenty years later I am struggling to learn the language and etiquette of this 'community-based' system. The current consultant, Dr Q, has been in post five years, but has had only essential and remote contact with myself and the few other GPs similarly interested and motivated. I once attempted to speak with him, about an obscured and worrying patient-situation: I hoped for the kind of dialogue I had, fruitfully and repeatedly, many years ago, with Dr M and his contemporaries. Dr Q's response was stiff in formality and cautious to the point of inertia. He quickly demonstrated (to himself) that there was little to discuss. As he spoke, I remembered old monochrome newsreels of the 1950s: the veteran Soviet Foreign Minister, Gromyko, and his stern monosyllabic camouflages, neutralising western journalists' eager questions. This opaque gravitas seemed both comic and threatening.

The threat is felt because the (Non) Spokesperson may foreshadow an enigmatic and concealed multitude, not a mere (and maybe) curmudgeonly individual. Silence can be interpersonal darkness, in highly vulnerable territory.

*

Other Practitioners are having similar problems. Like Dr K, a Local Medical Committee member. She is a warm-hearted, sharp-witted woman with a reputation for intelligent but humorous persistence. In an unscheduled encounter we briefly discuss my doldrums with local psychiatric services.

Her initial receptivity soon dissolves with gestures of thwarted aggravation. "It's hopeless," she summarises with testy terseness, "they're so boundaried and seem accountable only to their own management … I can't get any real dialogue from them, just organisational ripostes … I've given up …"

I think of Dr M's metaphor of the previous psychiatrists working in The Castle on the Hill, and how we have somehow, at great expense, replaced it with local armed garrisons of foreign soldiers, who speak only their own language. I share these evolutionary images with Dr K. We laugh heartily at this vignette of The Law of Unintended Consequences, but it is the manic, displacing laughter of doomed respite.

As our laughter falls away, I am aware of a sadness; a grieving, a realisation that valued activities and contacts are gone. Relinquished for those that seem (to me) to lead to such misalignment and derogated contact. Is the problem, mostly, that in my fortieth year of practice I am too rigid to mould to the cusp of change? Or is this more a cultural grief, for the passing of a collegial culture that was more responsive in its informality, pluralist and 'organic' in its growth. Replaced by a managed culture of sharply boundaried and structured multidisciplinary teams, themselves issuing and receiving 'information' and 'action plans'; where any 'development' is engineered and sanctioned by official diktat and now, increasingly, 'market forces'?

*

I try to get Amanda beyond her templated telephone 'management' of Tessa and I. I am becoming impatient. I feel obstructed by an armoured inflexibility. These colleagues seem immured and impermeable. Most worrying, they seem unstoppably confident in making remote, procedural decisions about a complexly troubled person who they have never met.

Clearly, there is little precedent, capacity or inclination to engage with me: an observant, thoughtful practitioner (I like to think) who has known the patient twenty years. I need to inject (my) reality into this surreal impasse. I can do this by talking collegueially with Dr Q. I ask to speak to him.

"Dr Q is very busy in meetings, all day … In any case, as I told you, the decision was taken as a Team."

Her crisp voice now seems edged with reprimand. I am being managed. I imagine the bright, brittle shell of a mollusc, a protective exo-skeleton. An 'executive persona'.

*

Thirty-five years ago I worked with Carl in a large victorian mental hospital. As young, trainee psychiatrists we enjoyed a friendly network of peers and older mentoring consultants. The ancient institution's heavy, forbidding architecture was, paradoxically, home to a warmly personalised 'village' within the NHS. In my two years there, friendly collegial relationships extended far beyond my closer professional 'family' (psychiatrists, psychologists, PSWs); I developed affable and effective alliances with art therapists, rehabilitation officers, the laboratory manager, even the hospital telephone switchboard operator. All these were known by name, face, voice, styles of banter. Reminiscing, Carl and I remember them with surprising precision. Beyond our individual memories, this says a great deal about that old institution and its connection to people.

Carl and I were mostly blessed by similar personal continuity and attention in our clinical apprenticeships. We both were guided by Consultants who (often) had known their patients for many years. This knowledge was likely to be quite as much 'in vivo' as 'in vitro'. Individuals were 'known' not just by questioning in the consulting room. Often they had been seen, over many years, in their homes, with parents, partners, children, friends, neighbours, even the (then) 'family' doctor. Our mentoring consultants thus taught us a kind of 'Field Psychiatry'. Here was a long time-span, and a wide matrix of human connections and understandings. By example as much as theoretical formulation, we learned to be imaginative about the unspoken, respectful of the complexity of attachments (including our own). We were gently shown creative discipline amidst inevitable uncertainties. Likewise, a pragmatic scepticism of the incompleteness of our consensual psychiatric language and tools. We discussed how many individual exceptions there are to our theoretical generalisations. "The more you see of somebody, the more of somebody you see" was an anchoring, guiding principle.

For many years, after he became senior, Carl continued this trajectory; he managed and delivered a service that got to know well its many kinds of sufferers, often over several years. For those whose problems were longstanding and variable, he was unhampered in his experienced choice of approach. In calm times, he would offer accessible, gentle interest. When trouble brewed, he could fast-track to a more interventive and urgent out-patient appointment. When serious trouble impacted, he would admit the patient, to be cared for by the staff he knew well; another part of his therapeutic family. Amidst the stresses and tensions inevitable in psychiatry, he grew a quiet love for the satisfactions of his role as a kind of pater familias and patient gardener. During these two decades, I did not hear him speak of 'Holistic Practice', but recognised the radiation of these values.

*

In recent times, Carl and I are talking of our individual and common travails. At this august stage of a diligent and creative career, he is disheartened and despondent. Not from his marathon contact with the anguished, but with the ever-tightening structures and strictures of management.

"I'm now just stuck in an Out-Patient Clinic, which is run by managers ... I can't, myself, make an appointment for a patient I've known for years: it has to be referred by the GP (who, increasingly, may not know the patient) and then be assessed for 'suitability' by the team (ditto) ... If my well-known patient may need admission, I have to send them to another team they don't know, because I no longer have beds ... and if it's decided they don't need admission there's yet another team (who probably don't know the patient ...) to look after them at home ... So, we have the Community Mental Health Team, The Emergency Psychiatric Clinic, The Home Treatment Team, The In-Patient Unit, The Early Discharge Unit, The Assertive

Outreach Team ... that's not all, and there's more on the way: shall I tell you?"

I raise my hands limply in surrender: my comprehension is coagulating.

He continues in angry jest:

"Well, if you don't understand it, or can't remember it all, what do you think it's like for patients who are dizzy with *their* distress, chaos or instability? Very often the most basic and important thing we can do for people is to provide a familiar and stable source of understanding, comfort and recognition; an accessible and humane form of asylum. I've tried to warn and remonstrate about how this complex multi-team approach leads to personal disconnection. It's not just frequently distressing; it's cumbersome, inefficient, and thus much more expensive. An aggressively defensive manager recently said to me: 'Our job, and your job, Doctor, is to make sure there is continuity within and between teams. It's the team, not the person. That way the Patient Journey is integrated ...' '*Integrated Patient Journey*': what a professionally self-referring shibboleth! I hope it makes the managers and planners feel calmer and better, because that's not the experience I usually hear from patients. With them, much of my work is about trying to soothe administratively torn connections. Imbue a sense of personal, durable and sensitive contact ... that's not easy when, at the same time, I am attempting to explain and apologise for a system that is (for them) recurrently unfamiliar, and thus (for them) incomprehensible and undependable.

"Yes, we talk of 'Agreed Care Plans' but these are usually *our* schematic actions, to which the craven patient will usually concur (or pretend to). Those who explicitly will not, are likely to evoke our subsidiary, often tendentious, diagnoses: the patient is 'non-compliant', 'chaotic', 'uncooperative' and so forth. I find these 'Care Plans' are much more prescriptive and authoritarian than the more informal, conversational ways you and I used for decades. It's only the clothing, the spun language, that illusion the democratic. More smooth deceits of Political Correctness!..."

Carl seems a little self-surprised by the size of this bolus of professional frustration, and the force, though ease, with which he has expelled it. Knowing my kindred experiences, we are, both, more emboldened than embarrassed.

How has a practitioner of Carl's calibre, experience, and personal qualities become so restricted, deskilled and impoverished in his work? I want to know the hidden organisational history.

"Carl. You've been the Senior Consultant at your hospital, the Clinical Director of your Trust, Regional Postgrad Tutor, Fellow of your Royal College ..." I pin the medals to his chest, and then ask: "Who are the people who designed such a system? How did they decide on this? Who did they ask? When? You must know these things ..."

My clustered questions are insistent, but softly spoken.

Carl looks disarmed and discomfited by them: shards of freshly realised but compromised ignorance.

"Ah!" I exhale, now canny in recognition. I imagine a stage-curtain descending. The Triumph of Bureaucracy-become-Culture: The Dictatorship of Everyone by No One.

"It's fiendishly clever", I say with affected, boyish lightness. "I mean, how can anyone ever undo it ...?"

*

We decide we cannot discern the persons behind the plans, those behind the unplanned drift into depersonalised care. Our attention turns now to more generic influences: culture, economics, new technologies, the media ... We rummage in this attic-full of tangled puppet strings, previously unheeded. Carl and I, veteran cohorts, rejuvenate our fading energies with regenerated language and questions.

"If you're writing about this new, skewed rigidification of Psychiatry, you really should include these undiscussed influences", Carl says.

"But there are so many, and they're so subtle ... the article will be far too long ..." I falter, daunted.

"Well, condense it and offer it as an Appendix. You can always write it up more fully, later," proffers Carl, saturated, succinct and prescriptive.

I agree. Herewith.

Ω

Appendix:

Current and recent influences displacing Person-Centred, Holistic Healthcare, especially in Psychiatry and General Practice. Some brief notes.

1. Industrialisation/Mass Production

Now determining influence in most human activities and their objects. May be the most important and difficult to counter. Leads to standardisation and pre-packaging. Loss of individual input: craft, attention and interest. 'Factory sizes' only: no bespoke. Difficult to prevent anomie. Best only when human variables are minimal, e.g. Cataract extraction, Vaccination, Acute and severe physical illness. Least good with complex, changeable processes and atypia. (As 2 +3)

2. A(na)tomisation

Medical Model = MM= best when dealing with localised physical macropathology. (Much less effective in other areas.) Psychiatric services now very dominated by MM. Anato-atomisation = AA = Multiplying and confining specialisations according to smaller body areas. e.g. General Orthopaedics ----- Hip/ Knee/ Shoulder etc. GI - Upper GI/ Hepatobiliary/ Colorectal etc.

AA and MM lead to limiting analogy of 'Mental Disorders' being generic 'states', rather than individual 'processes'.

AA and MM are structural and mechanistic models. Thus v. compatible with Industrialisation/ Mass Production/ Management Hegemony/ Goals and Targets (see later).

Recent massive attempts to mimic AA in Psychiatry, by mixing patient behaviour with organisational expedience, e.g. CMHT, Dual Diagnosis, Assertiveness Outreach, Eating Disorders, Alcohol Dependence, Emergency Psychiatric, Home Treatment, Early Discharge ... Medieval Theological Problem = How many Angels can sit on a single pin-head? Current NHS problem = How many Clinics can medicalise human anguish and be paid for by one PCT?

Such designed complexification generates its own problems. Akin to fitting a 117-speed gearbox to a vehicle: gears will tend to miss or jam, power is lost in propelling the larger bulk of machinery, which is much more expensive to produce ...

3. Computers and IT

Based on binary code: 0 or 1. Difficult medium for creative uncertainty. Algorithmic processes/choices coded as clear and definite. Incompatible with ambiguity, multiple meanings etc. Likely to lead to reification: Mental illness seen as a 'thing' rather than an organising concept for complex, evanescent processes: leads to Knowledge as a 'commodity' rather than 'activity'; a 'product', not a 'creation'.

4. We know how to work things, but not how things work

Objects of our use increasingly maintenance-free, disposable, sealed-for-life. A growing conundrum and syndrome in our Hi-Tech world. Few users now understand the innards of their car or computer. Leads to widespread mastery-without-understanding mindset. e.g. psychiatrist who follows 'correct' (decreed) 'Treatment Pathways', but has little understanding of/interest in the unique experience and 'innards' of each patient. Management without personal understanding.

5. NHS Commissioning: Territoriality and Commodification

Commissioning conceived (presumably) to tighten and sharpen working awareness and performance. Does it? Model derived from corporate competitive commerce. Many unintended side-effects: Practitioners frequently more boundaried = affiliation to Trusts' short-term, measurable, G & T (Goals and Targets) rather than patients' longer-term, less measurable, health and welfare. Increasing resources spent on window-dressing, PR/'Spin', legal process. Officious practice = adhering to 'Letter of the Law', not cleaving to values underlying it. Rules devoid of jurisprudence. G & T very compatible with MM + AA (above). Fosters competitive, territorial behaviour, rather than cooperative, collegial alliances.

6. Governmental Modelling: Less Conscious influences

a) Since 1997 the previous (New Labour) government has had more lawyers in Cabinet than any previous. Hence accelerated tendency to rules, regulations, prescribed procedures in most difficult human problem areas, especially Health and Social Care, Education. Intelligent and creative flexibility initially displaced, eventually proscribed.

b) In recent years a very influential senior Minister of Health[2] has been a Laparoscopic Surgeon. His expertise re: illness and treatments is via well-defined (mostly successful) procedures to very confined body areas. (Where MM and AA are most effective.) His perspective on planning and funding derives from these. Problem = if too dominant, leads to impoverishment of more holistic approaches. Especially important re: syndromes that are chronic, incurable, fluctuating or non-localisable = much (most?) of Elderly, Primary, Psychiatric Care. Much more than MM/AA required with these.

7. The Climbié-Clunis Factor:[3] The ratcheting of Defensive Practice

In our media-dense world, we now mass-produce and sustain interest in the most extreme enactments of 'madness' and 'badness', as never before. These sporadic horrors are rare, through perennial. New (and understandable) government initiatives to assert 'authority': systems for early identification and sequestration of perpetrators. 'Never again.' Resulting mass micromanagement is doubtfully effective. May be less effective, due to secondary inflexibility. Services dominated by 'worse case scenario' become anxiously and narrowly focused: like phobic patient with rigid and controlled relationships. Another analogy: the over-armoured medieval knight who cannot walk, mount his steed, or respond dextrously to attack, when it comes. Lesson: too much caution creates new hazards.

Practitioners strangulated by procedure lose capacity for reception, perception and reflection.

8. Not only but also: unintended multiplications and extrapolations

AA will tend to fragment holistic care and its long-enough healing attachments. Increasingly, ever more numerous and boundaried teams then have to be staffed and trained for. Trainees (who may provide most consultations) are then necessarily rotated more frequently between these many teams. Q: How will doctors learn about the power and subtlety of caring attachments? Are we already losing arts and crafts in these? How can the emotionally vulnerable connect, trust and heal by submitting to a carousel of professional 'strangers', united largely by the managerial designation of a team?

This discontinuity recently and coincidentally amplified by EC Working Hours legislation. 'Rationing' of working-time necessitates even more complex rotas and teams.

Epilogue: Distant Voices – Paradoxical Times

Intentions and consequences can be very different. In the early 1930s few realised how long and dense would be the shadow cast by the sinewy and virile youth of Totalitarianism. Giovani Gentile ghost writes for Mussolini, with Olympian righteousness, *The Doctrine of Fascism*:

"Anti-individualistic, the fascist conception of life stresses the importance of the State and accepts the individual only in so far as his interests coincide with those of the State, which stands for the conscience and the universal will of Man as a historic entity. It is opposed to classical liberalism which arose as a reaction to absolutism and exhausted its historical function when the State became the expression of the conscience and the will of the People ..."

About 75 years later in the National Health Service of our liberal democracy, Dr Steven Ford, a medical practitioner, writes to *The Independent* newspaper:[3]

'The thrust in the health field is towards the establishment of legions of meekly compliant, cloned health-droids with narrow spectra of competencies, tightly yoked by legally enforceable contracts, protocols and guidelines. The fate of patients in the new regime is to be parcelled into managerially tidy job-lots and auctioned off to the lowest bidder. Managerial and commercial skills are more highly valued and rewarded than clinical ones ...'

Few have claimed to design this new legacy, but many, already, are clearer about its effects. Whoever redesigns this redesign will have much to draw from.

*

'A mariner must have his eye on the rocks and sands, as well as on the North Star.'

Thomas Fuller MD, *Gnomoligia* (1732)

References and footnotes

1.   NHS expenditure shows an accelerated increase in the last two decades, far beyond any inflation. Statistics published in Hansard show this to be nearly 300% in the period 1995-2007 (c. 220% when inflation-adjusted). GDP fractional expenditure shows a similar trend in this period, from c. 6% to 8%. Some of this increase is due to factors inevitable, widespread and desirable, e.g. more people getting relief or cure from more conditions, greater longevity, more sophisticated and effective investigations, interventions and medications.

Psychiatric services share most of these. Where the new design of such services is exceptional is in its generation of complexity, with all the more and less obvious additional costs.

2.   Lord Ara Darzi

3.   Victoria Climbié was a child murdered by her aunt and partner in 2000. Christopher Clunis, known to be disturbed and labelled 'Paranoid Schizophrenia', murdered a stranger 'randomly' in 1992.

Both cases led to castigation of relevant professions (Social and Psychiatric Services respectively). Followed by demand for more management, supervision, documented procedures. 'Never again.' Major historical influences in current overgrowth of 'defensive practice'.

4. *The Independent*, Letters, 13/12/08
At the time of writing Tessa has been lost to contact. This followed my rejected referral. The connection seems significant, and I fear the gravity of the consequences. More positively, after many initiatives I have arranged a meeting with my CMHT.

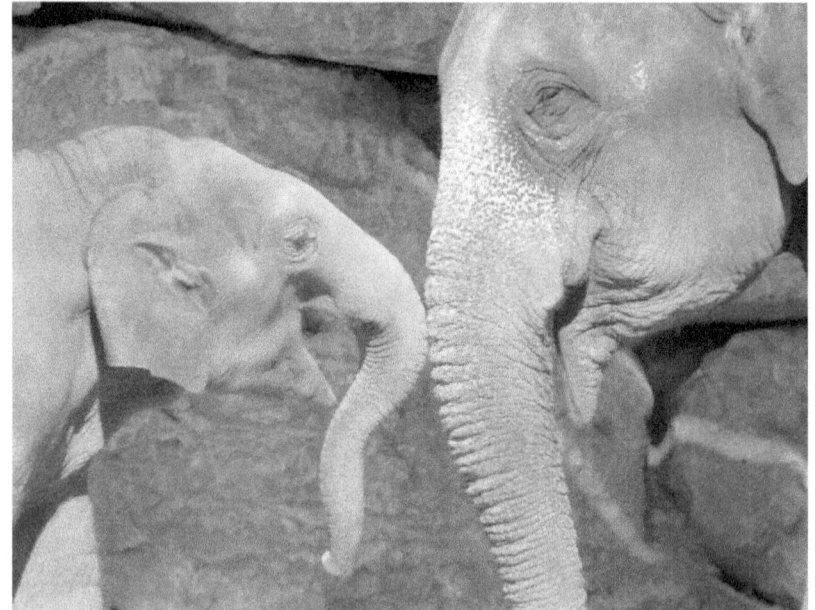

Why would Anyone Use an Unproven Therapy?

Treasures in the Mist: Another personal view

Not everything that can be counted counts. Not all that counts can be counted.

Albert Einstein, 1879-1955

Religion is regarded by the common people as true, by the wise as false, and by the rulers as useful.

Seneca the Younger, ca 4BC-65AD

Professor Edzard Ernst's 'Personal View'[1] is a short, robustly sensible piece. He leads us briskly along a much used path, pointing out how straying into surrounding, unscientific territory subjects us to the lures of fantasy, corruption and personal influence. The tarmacked path is smooth, firm, safe and even; the wilderness is unmapped, hazardous, disorienting. It is stalked by predatory creatures. Why would anyone choose to traverse this Wilder Ness?

I am reminded of many scientific-rationalist thinkers who pour easy scorn on religion: its tenets are absurdly unprovable, its conduct inconsistent, its basest expressions shockingly destructive. Why would anyone pursue irrational belief? But Ernst's rhetorical question is less simple than apparent. It spawns many beyond. Some are explored in this longer reply.

While his critique is importantly true, it is crucially incomplete. In particular, myth and fantasy are often harbingers of our most positive aspiration and inspiration. Belief in the transcendent and the transpersonal can be powerfully transformative, but only for the believer. Far from whimsy, these complex phenomena have been shown to be essential components in studies linking religious faith and health resilience,[2] and multifarious research into placebos.[3] Over several decades, repeated investigation identifies how the emotional state, the belief and faith of the sufferer, and the perceived quality of contact with the Healer, make critical differences in illness experience and outcome.[4]

115

Such interactional and transpersonal factors may be scientifically discerned generally, though with some difficulty. This cannot be said of the individual transmission and processing of such influences. Here we enter different and difficult territory: the 'art' of medicine and healing. Here are personal perceptions of experience and meaning. These are transmitted mainly intersubjectively, thus generating subtly unique language, metaphors and rituals.[5,6] Such personal factors can become quite as important as the impersonal science of biomechanism. Dilemmas arise, for it is only the impersonal, the generic, that are readily accessible to the organising code of our quantitative science. With all else we must suffice with other kinds of understanding and evaluation. Biomechanical Medicine has had dramatic successes in the last century. It is also readily understandable, reproducible and testable in ways often impossible with other forms of healing.

But the reach and strength of science is gravitated to the externally measurable: the sharpness of its definition fades as it enters the dappled realms of inner experience and the complexly interpersonal. Absence of (scientific) proof is not proof of absence. We must be wary that this potent and precise, but limited, world of Biomechanical Medicine is not overused, assuming a kind of regal hegemony. Some areas are not its natural territory.

We should be imaginative, therefore, about complexity and thus paradox. It is true that interpersonal healing (in contrast to the Orderly Ness of generic biomechanical treatment) is a Wilder Ness; obscure to scientific mapping. Ineluctably, as Ernst reminds us, more vulnerable to contamination by human folly, deception, greed or grandiosity. But what of its opposite pole? By analogy, arcane and ancient religious texts have led to those most disturbing and cruel perversions of 'righteousness' and superstition. Yet those same texts, very differently selected, have led to millions of undramatic quieting comforts for the anguished, humble acts of inclusion and kindness and (irrational?) faith and hope in our troubled and evanescent lives.

We can think of a genus of basic existential anxieties: primordially the chaotic meaninglessness of life; our mortality, our cosmic insignificance, and our ultimate alone-ness. How well we make positive sense of, or adjustment to, or defences against, these anxieties will have a determining effect on the basic quality of our lives. This is enacted through our relationships, our state of health and our response to illness, when it comes.[7,8]

Core biomedical practice does not address these inner workings. Religion and healing have many approaches, both explicit and inexplicit. The inexplicit are conveyed by metaphor and ritual. Such become the common currencies of healing. Thus, for example, healing 'procedures' involving touch or gaze may symbolically communicate to the sufferer recognition, inclusion and significance; all important requisites to palliation and recovery.[4] The procedure is a kind of language, but it can only be 'spoken' if both participants have congruent belief systems about the affliction.[6]

All this comprises something of the 'art' of healing and medical practice, and why it is so difficult to standardise, measure or mass-produce. Another important way of distinguishing and understanding these activities is to consider the source of resources: external and impersonal, or internal and (inter)personal. Prevailing biomechanical treatment exerts its influence via the former: by externally located agents – be they chemicals, manipulations, instruments, radiations, stents or sutures. Likewise, understanding and explanation are of an objective, generic and impersonal kind. Both are externally 'conducted'.

By contrast the many kinds of healing address and facilitate the individual's innate capacities of immunity, growth and repair: this is an 'induction' of internal resources. It is the product of interpersonal exchanges within a relationship field. Although induction may be individually powerful in-vivo, it is a protean, evaporative process, very dependent on individual attunement. In-vitro attempts to mass-produce or measure are left mostly with empty husks. Experience yields only external epiphenomena to measurement. Inductive healing can gestate only in the Wilder Ness: a conundrum for those health planners and managers who understand.

The film 'The Wizard of Oz' illustrates this fertile but paradoxical subterraneum of healing with charming simplicity. Each major character represents a universal human developmental task; the failure to address these leads to dis-ease or sickness. The Lion must find the courage to be himself (Identity); the Tin Man his heart for others (Love); the Scarecrow his own thoughts (Logos); and Dorothy a place of peace, acceptance and kinship: 'finding my way home' (Belonging). To re-own these they must achieve something that seems impossible to them as individuals: destroy the Wicked Witch of the West – the despair, nihilism and hatred that we can all harbour and inflict. They manage this communally, pursuing a shared belief in a myth: the all powerful Wizard of Oz. It is through faith in this mythical Other that they transcend their habitual (self-)limitation, subtly trance-formed, then transformed.

Dorothy, later, accidentally discovers that The Wizard is an unremarkable man operating a panoply of pyrotechnics to create such hypnotic charisma. Dorothy confronts him:

'You're a very bad man!' shouts Dorothy, through angry tears.

'No, I'm not a bad man. I'm a very good man. Just not a very good wizard ...' comes a faltering, apologetic explanation.

I am reminded of a recently retired bishop telling me that he had lost his faith, but had found verve in becoming a 'born again atheist'. With a further paradoxical garnish, he told me he still liked to attend church services.

'Why?' I asked, perplexed.

'Because it is the prayer that is transformative, whatever the fiction of the myth. Through prayer I find a kind of empowered humility, a sense of myself more clear and connected, though more transient. Through faith in something far beyond myself, I become less defined by my faults, frailties and inevitable mortality. I can now do without God, but not without prayer ...'

'How do you manage that: the one without the other?' I ask, again puzzled.

'Ah, well, you have to be a bishop first!' he replied with teasing wit and ambiguity.

After my amused bemusement had passed, I was left thinking how multilayered and meaningful his reply had been. Or was I imagining his encoded and askance wisdom? Was that a private myth, of mine? In any case, this contact induced in me a burgeoning constellation of new thoughts and connections: I was enlivened, enriched and energised. A small incident, but I reflected on how this offered a microcosmic example of the questions we face with both healing and prayer. How do we even begin to measure, manage or mass-produce such subtle life-exchanges, such treasures in the mist? Do we need a Yellow Brick Road?

*

We can be absolutely certain only about things we do not understand.

Eric Hoffer. *The True Believer* (1951)

References and notes

[1] Ernst, E. Why would anyone use an unproven or disproven therapy? A personal view *Journal of the Royal Society of Medicine* 2009; 102: 452–53

[2] Frank, J *Persuasion and Healing*. New York: Schocken, 1972

Frank, J *Psychotherapy and the Human Predicament.* New York: Schocken, 1978
  Frank, a Professor of Psychiatry at John Hopkins Medical School, was a prodigious academic researcher and writer for several decades. He demonstrated the pathogenic influence of alienation and despondency. As a corollary, and their institutions. He showed, too, how these placebo effects could all be reversed by pessimism, mistrust and negatively-experienced attachments: the 'Nocebo' effect.
  Frank's work is equally impressive in its breadth, depth, meticulousness and clarity. The above two books offer the most accessible introduction.

[3] Ibid.
Zigmond, D. Mother, Magic or Medicine? The Psychology of the Placebo *British Journal of Holistic Medicine* 1984; 1:113–9
  The paper provides a brief survey of placebo research as well as providing some explanations from developmental and social psychology.

[4] Frank, J (1972), op cit; Frank J (1978), op cit

[5] Balint, M. *The Doctor, his Patient and the Illness*. London: Pitman, 1957

  Balint's informal, qualitative study was of encounters between General Practitioners and their patients. Amidst his clarifications was the importance of the inter-subjective in medical practice, which has become increasingly defined and confined by an objective view and language. He explored the different kinds of diagnostic and therapeutic opportunities that were possible from this interpersonal perspective, as well as the perils that followed its neglect.
  Due the difficulty (?impossibility) of standardising, regulating or mass-producing this approach, it has been responded to with bewilderment, indifference or hostility by, first, contemporary health

planners and economists and, then, managers and practitioners. In this author's view, the consequent loss of 'emotional literacy' to the cultures of General Practice and Psychiatry, is grievous: therapeutically, economically and experientially.

[6)] Zigmond, D. Three Types of Encounter in the Health Arts: Dialogue, Dialectic and Didactism. *British Journal of Holistic Medicine* 1987; 2:68-81

A short paper considering how practitioners and patients jointly process experience and language in different kinds of transactions. These confer power, agency and responsibility in very contrasting ways. The origins of these and the consequences of misappropriation and misalignment are illustrated and explained.

[7)] Balint, M (1970). *Treatment or Diagnosis. A Study of Repeat Prescriptions in General Practice.* London, Tavistock

Another of Balint's substantial, small scale, quantitative researches, over many years. Explores how many illness behaviours and their medical responses are best understood as ritualistic, encoded communications, which both doctors and patients often resist decoding. As with (6), above, now much neglected, with considerable loss of personal types of understanding.

Quite as important, he showed the therapeutic effect of: feeling re-engaged with peers, having an explanation congruent with native beliefs, a sense of positive personal agency and some evidence of its success. Pre-requisite to these were faith, trust and positive attachment to healers and Another of Balint's substantial, small scale, quantitative researches, over many years. Explores how many illness behaviours and their medical responses are best understood as ritualistic, encoded communications, which both doctors and patients often resist decoding. As with (6), above, now much neglected, with considerable loss of personal types of understanding.

[8)] This was well illustrated in an NHS project in the late 1980s. An Alternative/Complementary Medicine Clinic was set up for GPs and Hospital Practitioners to refer to. The results, in terms of therapeutic results, and even attendance, were poor. The Alternative Practitioners were equally dismayed and puzzled: they had abundant good evidence of much better results in their private practices.

In this author's view procedures might be the same in the two settings, transactionally they were very dissimilar. In Private Practice both patient and practitioner are likely to assume convergent values, expectations, maybe myths. There is a shared 'language'. In the NHS, where a third party organises the dyad by referral, there is less likelihood of such a 'match', and thus no occult 'common-language'. These exchanges are thus less receptive to the possibilities of 'induction'.

The hypothesis here is that it is the encrypted 'communication' that is therapeutic, not the procedure per se.

[Experience from Author's own practice.]

Ω

Publ. by *Journal of Holistic Healthcare* Vol. 7 Issue 2 Sept. 2010

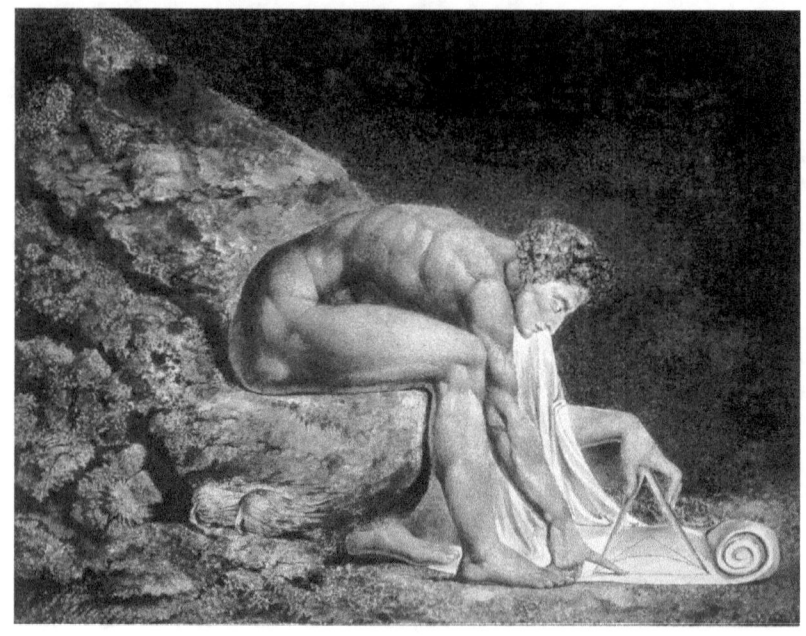

William Blake – *Isaac Newton* 1805

Idiomorphism
the Lost Continent

How diagnosis displaces
personal understanding

Introduction and summary

In understanding of the non-human world, our scientific procedures and 'objective' observation and generic clustering serve us well. But human complexity renders such presumptions much less reliable: motivation, protean states of (un)consciousness, encoded behaviours and communications, concealed diversities – all such phantoms are signifiers of the human condition; and all are frequently elusive and impenetrable to our usual scientific endeavours.

Publicly provisioned healthcare is now largely designed and guided by a new cultural convention: 'Evidence Basis'. This is anchored to science whose competence is rooted in the impersonal. While this often works well in dealing with clear physical disease – 'structural pathology' – it becomes adversely inadequate with other kinds of distress. It is these 'functional disturbances' – dis-ease – that comprise the subtlest challenges to healthcare. Our understanding and response to this world of human complexity, paradox and chimera needs very different, though complementary, skills. The illustrating vignettes in this article are authentic and typify what is common in primary care. In psychiatry and psychology it is the subterraneum, though now increasingly, and hazardously, disregarded.

How do we respond?

*

'Though all men be made of one metal, yet they be not cast all in one mould'

John Lyly Euphus, *The Anatomy of Light* (1579)

'Every man is more than just himself: he also represents the unique, the very special and always significant and remarkable point at which the world's phenomena intersect, only once in this way and never again.'

Herman Hesse, *Prologue to Demian* (1979)

A. Idiomorphism – People's stories. Samples from primary care. End: Week 1

1. Cathy

Age 63, Cathy has suddenly looked older, since she found her husband, Bob, collapsed and dead in the bathroom. A stalwart and uncomplaining man, his life suddenly ended; a mortality shocking for its lack of warning. The coroner had judged it due to a massive heart attack.

Dr R had had only light and infrequent, though amiable, contact with Bob over many years. Cathy's many encounters with her doctor had been very different. Twelve years ago she had discovered Bob in a secret, flirtatious tryst with a younger woman. Theirs was a long marriage, blighted by infertility; for decades they compensated with affectionate care and companionship. Until this quaking portent of infidelity and abandonment.

Cathy had responded with a primitive and punitive maelstrom of explicit and encoded emotion. Fear, grief, rage, despair all fed into her abject and retributive broth of distress of body and mind. How could either she, or he, be motivated or permitted to go on living in the wake of such betrayal? Earlier Dr R had feared explosive or implosive catastrophe. After six years he felt safer; like a clergyman suggesting, nurturing and guiding buds of forgiveness. Cathy now sustained a warily melancholic marital bond with Bob: 'I love him but I won't tell him, or allow him too close ... he has to sleep on the sofa, doctor'.

Two days after she finds his just-deceased body, warm but unbelievably still on the bathroom floor, she seeks out Dr R. She is ushered in, kindly, by the receptionist as an end-of-surgery 'Emergency'. She is almost mute with shocked intensity, choked and blinded with tears. Dr R knows he cannot hurry – he has to lean far forward to hear her barely expressed voice: ' I thought I heard a "crump" but I wasn't sure ... I waited a minute, then went in and found him ... I think I could have saved him, if I'd gone immediately ... So it's my fault: if it weren't for me, he'd be alive ... I don't think I can live without him ... Does he know that, doctor? ... Do you?'.

*

2. Amir

When Amir first came, he could not talk of his hurts, his shame, his well of sadness, his furnace of fury. Only slowly has Dr R understood the exhausting struggle Amir has to endure and bear alone. Amir is a large-framed, but compliant and placatory man. His story, which Dr R has always believed, was largely made and smashed by others. His arranged marriage in India, to Kalpur, twenty years ago, had been largely fertilised and conceived by their two prominent and dominant families in a small Kashmiri town. After their arrival in London fifteen years ago, Amir had felt blessed with Kalpur, their new country and the birth of three daughters. Social and biological fate seemed to be gently smiling on them all.

Back in Kashmir, destructive troubles were hatching that he was not party to, did not understand and could never influence. Like a terrible storm, these troubles would quickly devastate his life's achievements and plans. In the North of Kashmir their two families had fallen into a primitive and internecine feud.

Kalpur, perplexedly paralysed and then controlled by the most commanding gravitational force, turned on, then ejected her husband from the family group.

When he first came to see Dr R, his distress was so raw, intense and beyond his usual vocabulary, that he could hardly speak. His demeanour told Dr R much more: his sagged, leaden gait; tearful eyes, avoiding contact, yet conveying fear and shame; a voice defeated, yet still apologetic; smart clothes, now crumpled.

From this fragile and inchoate tangle Dr R had to be delicate and patient in constructing a story – Amir's 'History' – explaining not only his immediate symptoms – his dis-ease – but also his massive losses: of marriage, fatherhood, family, home and occupation – his alienation.

After Amir's faltering and pained initial meeting with Dr R, the doctor had thought Amir's risk and distress were so high he should see a psychiatrist urgently. This was arranged with seamless rapidity. The assigned contact was more problematic: Amir later said 'they [the Psychiatric Team] just kept asking all these questions about "voices", and whether I really wanted to kill myself … so much, so many questions! … I couldn't really speak, or even think…' Amir refused to return to them.

Dr R thought of the old term for psychiatrist – 'Alienist' – and how this connoted a practitioner skilled in the art of healing torn or withered connections – with one's Self, Others, the world around. Dr R thought that these current Alienists were themselves alienated, at least from Amir and *his* alienation.

About a year later Amir gazes at Dr R, now with warmth, sorrow, calmness and deliberation. 'If you hadn't understood me or my situation then I wouldn't be alive now', he says with quiet, economic gratitude. Dr R experiences some glow of satisfaction. It is shared evidence, and private recognition, of his piloting such tempestuous seas. But he is also disquieted; harried by a wider concern: if he had not undertaken this, who would?

*

3. Clare

Clare was tormented, feared she could not understand her feelings, nor be understood. 'Am I going mad, doctor?...' Twelve years ago, her relationship with Danny had finished with ugly and menacing cacophony, leaving her alone with two small sons. Danny had always been demanding and jealous of her attention, and could not accept his new role of father, with all its compromises and deferred gratifications. Danny's second act of drunken violence decided Clare's finishing their relationship, though not her yearning or grief. After a dangerous and tangled period of threats, court appearances and injunctions, Danny retreated. Clare was left to complete the long and lonely voyage of single motherhood. Danny has not been seen for years.

Clare has heard that Danny is in prison, for another violent crime. Her sons, Sean, 15, and Craig, 17, have also heard. She has been having problems with Craig's increasing adolescent anger and intimidation; now it is worse: 'Craig's now very tall: taller than Danny ... he gets so angry, I often think he's possessed by some kind of demon ... he stands over me, his voice so loud and hard: the worst thing is that he sounds and looks to me just like Danny, all those years ago ... My feelings are so mixed-up: I become really scared, and at the same time often hate Craig, for being so like Danny ... I feel resentful and then so guilty ... How can I feel these things, as his mother? ... Can you understand all this, doctor?'

Dr R thinks this is a rhetorical question, for which she is seeking his reassurance and validation: she would not have entrusted him with 'all this' if she felt he had not understood. Dr R muses on understanding this understanding: how it has arisen from years of unstructured and unscheduled contacts, each adding to a growing bond of trusting familiarity, each enabling thoughts to be clarified, feelings to be verbalised, connections to be seen. Like a gardener, he could not use his skills to command these processes; only encourage, protect and nourish what might emerge.

*

4. Alf

Alf carries his 82-year-old, tall frame with remarkable uprightness, discipline and pride. He has been wearing a similar brass-buttoned navy-blue blazer since Dr R first met him in the 1970s, but it never looks worn. Despite this mien of well-kempt fortitude, Alf now looks pale and unwell. He crosses the room with slow, frail caution. As he sits down Dr R is struck by the depleted timbre of his voice, the deadness of his gaze. Alf had come with such heralding signs of depression many times and years before when, at least, his physical health was then robust.

Dr R had also known Alf's brothers. All four had a similar manner of intelligent, diligent courtesy. All had followed their father's occupation in the London Docks. Remarkably, all had remained unmarried and, at some time, all had been treated at the old Victorian Mental Hospital. Dr R can remember mechanically-typed letters from the 1960s, documenting how all (and the deceased father, and father's father, and father's brother) had suffered from 'Periodic Familial Melancholia', later 'Recurrent Endogenous Depression'. Dr R had been encouraged by how their afflictions became more manageable as the medications had improved. A fascinatingly clear constellation illustrating 'biological psychiatry', Dr R had said several times to his students.

Despite his current bleakness, it seems important for Alf to have this contact with Dr R:

'My life seems so empty, so meaningless … My brothers have all died and now I have no family at all … My Chinese neighbour doesn't speak English, or even know my name … Now I've got prostate cancer, I've never felt so alone: you're

now the only person that's known me, from all those years ago
…'

He pulls himself up in his chair, his voice a little stronger:

'All my usual symptoms have come back, really badly. So, I remembered what you said last time, and yesterday increased my [antidepressant] tablets. I know there's nothing else for you to do, doctor, but I just thought you'd want to know … Shall I come back in a fortnight, so you can see how I am …?'

Alf, like his brothers, has never obstructed more personal exploration, though never benefited from such efforts either. Dr R has little to do but be mindful and respectful of the subtext. He ponders how apparently simple is his task, yet how important it is for Alf. Any attempt to diminish or delete this humble but subtle role would, very likely, have tragic consequences. The paradoxical skill lies in recognising the complexity of the simple.

*

5. Tom

Tom's normally aquiline, handsome features are shockingly obscured. His left eye is almost closed by grey and purple swelling. Above it a normally elegantly arched eyebrow has been torn, now stitched and encrusted by dried blood. A domed grey-brown bruise on his left forehead sits astride this ugly asymmetry.

Tom is unable to offer his usual playful smile to Dr R: he is hurt and hurting. 'I was Gay-Bashed … they came from behind, four of them, maybe five: I couldn't see and didn't stand a chance … I know who they are. The Police want my injuries recorded, and I just wanted to tell you anyway…'

A year ago Tom had come with a less visible but equally distressing pain. His father had died very rapidly from an unsuspected but evidently virulent malignancy. Tom had never had a satisfactory bond with his father: he had experienced him as critical, harsh and controlling. Tom's mother was lovingly collusive with Tom about his homosexuality, but it was never openly acknowledged with father: an unexploded bomb.

Tom, now mid-thirties, has built himself a stable and positive life: good friends, a loving partner and a meticulously orderly occupation as an Air Traffic Controller. But there is a painful gap where there was no loving father: his grief is not for the father he lost, rather the father he never had. Dr R, during Tom's fresh grief, had talked with him a few times of such things, helping him through this raw ravine. Dr R was aware of his likely role, as an older man: the father who listens, includes, accepts. The father Tom never had. Dr R thought Tom clearly realised this, though they spoke of it only lightly and elliptically.

Tom's bruised humiliation seems lightened by Dr R's inspection, witness and then suggestion that he returns in a week 'to see how things are settling'. Dr R thinks that Tom understands the meaning of this connecting and containing healing ritual.

'Thanks, Doc: you're a rock!', he says with a brave lopsided smile and an offer of affectionate banter.

*

As Dr R finished his Friday evening surgery, he thinks of Cathy, Amir, Clare, Alf and Tom – and others, too, he has seen that day – each a mixture of the universal and the unique. For each struggles for personal connection, meaning, definition, safety, comfort, recognition or belonging. Lost or foundering in the struggle, each may be diagnosed as having 'Anxiety' or 'Depression' – these are easily packaged: elementary clusters in an inevitably crude science of distress. Yet it is perceiving the uniqueness of each individual and each consultation that has most sustained, for many years, Dr R's interest, engagement and Élan Vital. This is the Art and, Dr R has long thought, the heart of healing. Here, in this fragile, often elusive but powerful space within and between persons, is where compassionately imaginative contact can grow its most prized fruit.

*

B. The Generic – Cluster, convention and code. Start: Week 2

It is late Monday morning and Dr R has cleared the rest of the day to attend a large professional area meeting: Plans for Commissioning Mental Health Services. Before he goes, he steels himself to read another administrative obelisk: a lengthy and didactic diktat from the National Institute of Clinical Excellence (NICE): 'The Management of Anxiety and Mood Disorders'. The format is familiar: first the awakening warning of how large is the problem and its cost in personal, financial and organisational terms; then the complex problem is broken down into functional or administrative subcomponents; finally each is delegated or despatched, via serial towers of bullet points and forests of algorithms. Implicitly it is only the parts that matter; the whole becomes an irrelevant abstraction. Dr R, heeding some internal voice of higher authority, deflects his own objections and instead disciplines his attention until the end of this document of instruction. As he does so he feels his mind constrict, his energy deplete. An unbidden childhood memory comes into his mind: an image of a Primate confined to a small bare cage in a city zoo.

What will this afternoon's meeting bring?

*

Dr S is addressing the serried ranks of higher echelon healthcare workers. His manner is courteous, amiable but commanding: a public school headmaster pep-talking his staff. He makes clear how important it is that clear diagnoses are made, so that the correct care-pathways can be followed. This can be done by filling in relevant questionnaires and algorithms that clarify, validate and quantify diagnosis: the nature and severity of the complaint thus becomes defined precisely. This yields a clear path – necessary not just for more scientific research, but also more effective treatment and then commodification. Commissioning will be expedited: more funding can be garnered. Thus, increasingly, mental illnesses will be diagnosed, containerised, despatched, streamed, managed and marketed: like procedures in physical illness now, in the new NHS economy.

The audience looks, Dr R thinks, mostly acquiescent, but not engaged: semi-slumped to obediently receive these new notions of authority. Dr R is thinking how these devices of cluster, convention and code are predicated on generic similarities, but become inimical to his personal understanding. They help him little with the complex dances he must improvise to help others find courage, heal and grow. How do we address such limitless human complexity and variation with sense and sensibility; to accurately understand each person and their maybe-similar-but-always-unique difficulties? The *Generic* is the accessible territory for planners, statisticians, economist and managers: but it is the *Idiomorphic* that often most helpfully guides the practitioner – to make personal sense with *this* person, *now*. When the Generic and Idiomorphic seem largely congruent, there may be few problems. When they are not, which is frequently, the art, skill and judgement of the practitioner are more tested.

Dr R, over decades, had attempted to repair the damage done to many patients where the generic medical or psychiatric diagnosis was expounded and executed with such unchallenged authority that any personal perspective or meaning became completely displaced. This management-without-personal-understanding was rarely beneficial and often harmful: it added to the sufferer's sense of alienation, passivity and disempowerment. Such are the perils of overusing the Medical Model. Dr R now listens to Dr S's plans for increasing the hegemony of the Generic-Medical-Psychiatric phalanx, driving its 'authority' deeper into the human wilder-ness; a realm where more fluid and delicate understanding is required. He fears not just for the fate of his patients, but his own professional integrity.

Dr R speaks out and attempts to condense his notions and concerns with courtesy but conviction. Dr S is also courteous, but appears distracted, bemused and uncomprehending. While Dr R wonders whether this is a cannily disingenuous ploy, he looks around at his colleagues. Some are looking towards him, smiling tentative encouragement. Others gaze down and away, averse to any possible discordance, especially with authority. The remainder remain immobile and impassive: bystanders. Dr S urbanely moves the meeting on: 'Any other questions?'.

As the proceedings close, several delegates approach Dr R, to offer nervous support and confederation. One is Dr T, a formally dressed, middle aged, softly spoken man. He looks over his shoulder and says, with a quietness bespeaking conspiracy: 'I'm really pleased you said all that ... I don't think I'd have the courage, even if I could find the words'.

*

Forty years ago Dr R read a, then seminal, book by a maverick, elderly Hungarian psychoanalyst, Michael Balint. It was titled 'The Doctor, his Patient, and the Illness', and enriched the working lives and relationships of hundreds of General Practitioners, for a generation. Balint met regularly, for many years, with a small group of GPs, building up portraits and understandings of the personal and interpersonal subtext of their medical practice: the unexpressed or hidden world of feelings, impulses or thoughts that lay behind the diagnoses, procedures and technical utterances – the generic. This type of *qualitative* research was never officially sanctioned or funded. It has been long supplanted by *quantitative* studies, conditionally financed and committee-endorsed. But Balint's informal research path had powerful cultural and educational effects: by freeing doctors to explore the idiomorphic, Balint enabled these practitioners to find new types of meaning and understanding in their encounters with the distressed and disrupted. They found themselves more able to heal, as well as treat: most reported much deeper work satisfactions. Such were Dr R's early mentors.

But Balint's influence was in a time of unwrapping: a time of adulterated disciplines and feral philosophy: an era whose health practitioners were often insighted and incited by such creative deconstructionists as Laing, Szasz and Illich.

There are now no such luminaries to excite professional human curiosity: professional motivation is now engineered by a financially induced system of NICE guidelines, QOF points, goals and targets, and an endless rash of algorithms. Dr R is now struggling to find intellectual oxygen and human sustenance in this period of near-ubiquitous tight wrapping and containerisation. It is not just his supermarket that standardises, unit-packs, film-wraps and bar-codes natural products for managed distribution. He is working for a healthcare service that intends to do the equivalent with much higher and more sentient life forms. He thinks of Cathy, Amir, Clare, Alf and Tom ...

How do we respond?

'The young man knows the rules: the old man knows the exceptions.'

Portuguese proverb

Ω

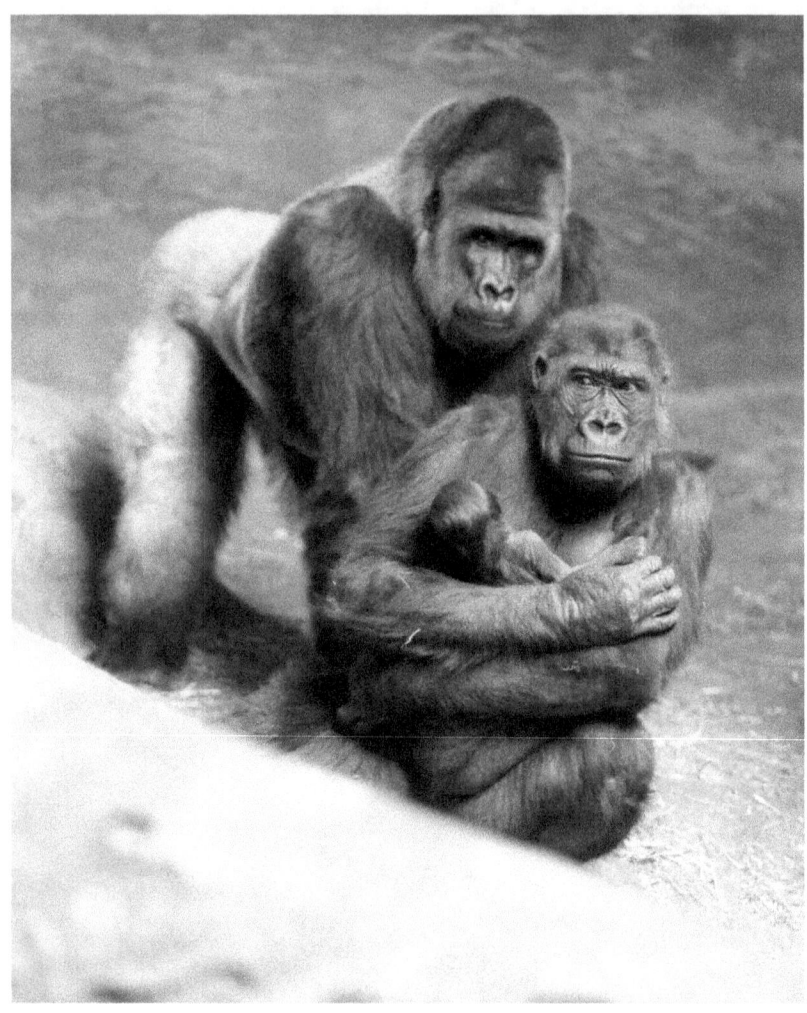

Resolved or Abandoned?

Irresponsibly lost Transference:
a professionally embarrassed tale

June 1980

"COME IN! ... JUST COME IN!!" My head is crowned with shampoo-lather and I shout through a haze of rising steam. I hoped that the open door would transmit my hollered voice to the front door that I had deliberately left ajar. I was expecting my teenaged stepson: he did not have keys.

The shrill ringing of the doorbell paused, then resumed. Flustered and irritated, I boomed my imperative message even louder through the bathroom steam. Surely, now he could hear.

Again, the high pitch of the doorbell drills the air. Why does he not let himself in? Realising now that direct action was needed to resolve this ambiguity, I clambered, hurried and harried, from my bath. I wrapped the closest, but small, towel round my nether regions, and, dripping and squinting, descended the twilit staircase to the half-open front door. The pattered trail of bath water was joined by thin, grey rivulets of shampoo from my mid-washed hair.

I pulled with angry impatience at the front door, to open it fully. Shouted banter at my stepson, attributing impaired hearing and intelligence, completed my unsighted greeting.

*

On the other side of the door was not my stepson. It was Elizabeth.

*

We both stared and blinked: a hiatus of dislocated incredulity. I, for forgetting (or 'forgetting') the unusual appointment time she had requested; I had agreed to this, as a 'one-off'. She, for now seeing this previously contained and impeccably professional young man in such feral and primitive disarray.

*

Elizabeth was a refined, intelligent, insighted, but painfully inhibited woman. Twenty years older than I, she had almost entirely negative memories of her Edwardian father: remote, humourless, austere, rigid, inexpressive. His barren, dark influence shadowed her life for sixty years. I, too, became an extension of that shadow. Despite my best efforts to bridge the gap, she remained ill at ease. My proffered utterances may have clarified, but did not console. She came assiduously, but I had to imagine beyond her carapace.

*

Both Elizabeth and I were struck immobile for several seconds: time to adjust our eyes, then our minds, to our respective shocks. The door had been opened: views had changed, forever.

My reaction was the more predictable: I attempted to rapidly cluster sincere apology, embryonic explanation, reassurance and a pragmatic, emergency plan – for her to return in thirty minutes, when I would be suitably attired and prepared. I improvised a pitch of tone, between professional gravitas and friendly-fallible.

*

Elizabeth's reaction was less predictable, and certainly more interesting. She laughed. First with discrete softness, but soon with raucous warmth. It was not the harsh, abrasive laughter of triumph or mockery, but the peeling, joyous, contagious laughter of shared realisation, relief and release. The laughter of unanticipated enlightenment. For her, my chaos had humanised us both. For me, her laughter had freed us both.

*

This perilously comic error had serious, yet benign, consequences. Elizabeth's dense and massive father-transference had been blown away, with a speed and finality that were probably impossible with careful, systematic therapy. The changes spread far beyond the therapy room, too. She reported a blessed shock-wave re-configuring all her important relationships.

Some months later she and I recalled these events and their surprising evolution. She drew on her background in literature and offered me an oblique observation of GK Chesterton: "Humour can get under the door while seriousness is still scrabbling at the lock."

August 2011

This transformative comedy of errors occurred more than thirty years ago. How did it change me? On a superficial level, I check my diary more carefully: I am more vigilant to possible error. More deeply, and complexly, it opened my mind to the (often) paradoxical nature of human difficulty, struggle and change. Experience is not just a living process: it is an evolving one, too – it develops new and unpredictable forms. Hence, there is little science of the individual's metabolism of meaning.

Would I try it again, now, as a procedure? Certainly not: I am far too orthodox…

$$\Omega$$

An edited version is included in *The Business of Therapy: How to Run a Successful Private Practice* by Pauline Hodson (2012), Open University Press, McGraw Hill

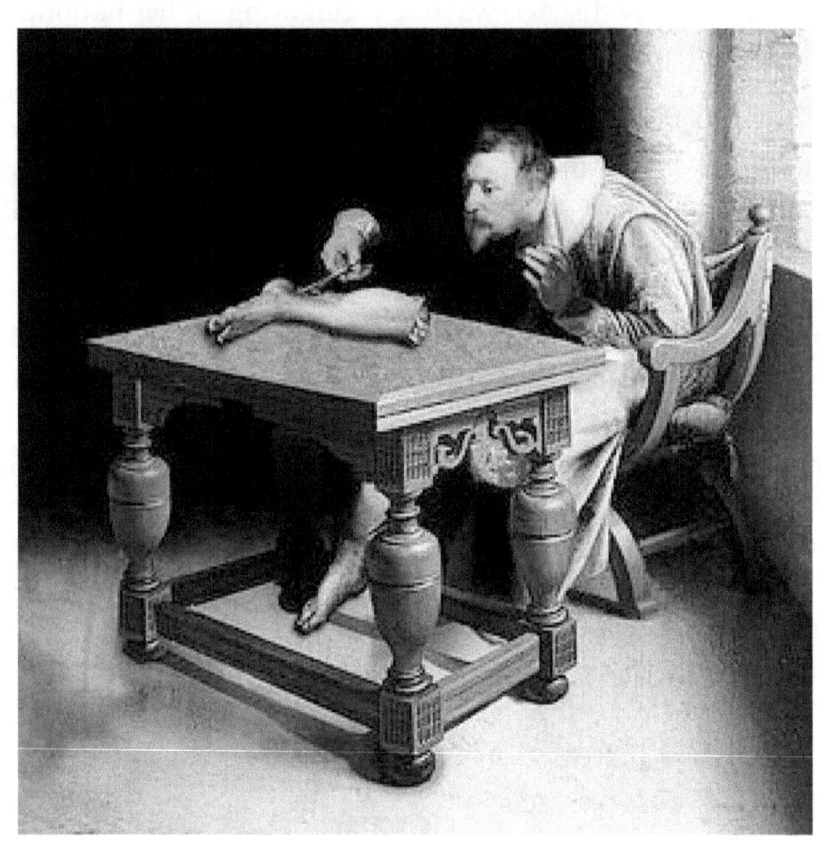

Philip Verheyen dissecting his amputated leg Anonymous 1675

Sense and Sensibility

The danger of Specialisms to holistic, psychological care

Increasing specialisation in healthcare is often equated with progress. Yet often, though subtly, specialisation is destructive of valuable aspects of healthcare. This article explores this theme, using the example of Specialist psychologists working with Acute Mental Illness.

'Ten Lands are sooner known than one man'

Yiddish proverb

Prologue

The use of technical language and understanding to designate and remedy the entire span of distress presented to healthcare workers is partly indispensible and inevitably expands. A burgeoning of specialisms follows. Each of these, to survive, needs to develop its own distinctive language and models. The benefits of these, in some areas, have been dramatic and transformative. But such benefits become much more doubtful when problems are not primarily physical. This short essay is a response to another article proposing that the acutely mentally ill might be better served by a further elaboration of specialist services and vocabularies. The counter-argument, proposed here, is that such developments, when misplaced, often take us *away* from the kinds of personal engagement and understanding that are most likely to be healing and helpful. Neglect or abandonment of these may be inadvertent, but are insidious and growing threats to the quality and integrity of personal care.

As we get older, and when our turn comes, we are grateful for the sharp, narrow focus of specialisation. For the failing heart or eye, we welcome the territorially different skills, applied with strict topographic attention, mandating distinctions between cardiac valve and coronary artery, the lens cataract and diabetic retinopathy. We may challenge the competence of the specialist, but not his speciality.

We can call this process of progressive division of healthcare into smaller and smaller foci of activity 'Anatoatomization' (AA). This term signifies its derivation from the Medical Model (MM), a fault-in-the-machine paradigm. This, too, is based on anatomy and physiology; like foundation stones to a column of medical specialities, each successive layer becoming increasingly refined and confined.

MM and AA work so well in certain areas, that challenges rarely occur. The more anatomically located or acute the problem, the more true this is. Medical and surgical emergencies serve well as examples of near inviolability.

The *science* involved in such (MM and AA) defined activities proceeds via our conventions of clustering our observations by similarities: generic patterns. In contrast, there are other aspects to healthcare where, instead, the *art* discerns and navigates our innumerable (and less measurable) human variables; the personal and subjective – the dissimilarities that make each of us who we are. Such art and science are tensely counter-poised, but often symbiotic: an eternally recurrent test of balance and judgement for practitioners.

MM and AA, then, have well earned and well based pragmatic hegemony when dealing with physical disease: solid-state pathology. Adam Smith's doctrine of Division of Labour is here on very workable territory. But this hegemony is extended, then overextended, to other areas, and for other reasons. The language and model imply powerful blessings: for authority, definition, standardisation and measurability. This apparent conferral of clarity and control seems irresistible to planners, economists and managers. Adoption is eager and rapid. Scientifically sounding phrases then expediently bolster the language of governance: it becomes difficult to distinguish the scientific from the scientistic. Thereafter, in a cascade effect, these flow down as a kind of didactic Esperanto, instructing and defining the caring professions. The result is the 'medicalisation' of almost any problem of experience, learning, adjustment or relating. There are, too, larger cultural forces at work. For we, in our advanced industrial society, now rarely encounter the unpackaged and unlabelled. Our minds are now rendered disconcerted and distrustful by the feral and undesignated. Packaging becomes symbolic of safety.

Our medicalisation of non-anatomical problems can certainly (if transiently) seem to quell complex human uncertainties by a kind of rhetorical aura. Sometimes this is followed by real and sufficient help. Often, though, it turns specious from its assumed clarity and authority. This is because medicalised understanding is confined to generic patterns. It does not extend to individual struggle, evolution or meaning: the 'idiomorphic'. Within the ill-defined compass of Psychiatric and General Practice, in particular, practitioners who become unreceptive to the idiomorphic will miss and misconstrue much that they encounter. While 'treatment' may depend largely on objectification (MM), and thus be well-served by specialisation (AA), 'healing' runs counter to these: it requires approaches that are holistic, personal and interpersonal. Broadly speaking, treatment represents the convergence of 'science', healing the divergence of 'art' in encountering human distress.

I recently read an article: 'Where does Psychology fit in Acute Mental Health Wards?'.[1] The writing was, I thought, a solidly competent contribution to the current thinking and culture of psychiatry and medically orientated psychology. But I was struck, and increasingly interested, by a central axiom: one deriving from, and then contributing to, our increasing tendency to an errant, fragmented specialisation. It was that psychology is a naturally divisible activity from, though an optional ally to, psychiatry. This premise produces more difficulties than it solves, for such assumed divisions will seriously obstruct possibilities of holistic personal understanding and care. This poses particular hazards throughout psychiatry and medical practice. What kind of artless practice will remain if we do not include skilful address

---

[1] McGowan, John and Hill, Rosalind (2011) 'Where does psychology fit into acute mental health wards?'. Submission to The Psychiatrist

of the unobvious and the unspoken? The article's designated problem of acute mental illness, in particular, represents such inchoate territory: the breakdown of an individual's functioning, integration and identity. What healing we can muster attempts to counter this with varieties of holistic reparation: good continuity and quality of personal contact are elemental and essential. To be personal, such contact must be bespoke and dextrous: this requires a wide repertoire of skills offered *in-vivo*. This kind of engagement is always a delicate dance and easily stymied,[2] for example, by any attempt to fragment personal suffering into academically abstracted sub-components, each to be sub-contracted *in-vitro*. (Presumably, eventually, algorithms would be designed to command this!)

More basically, in most of our many forms of interpersonal care, we are best served when we are imaginatively receptive. For human vulnerability usually ushers a complex of unarticulated fears and encoded needs. To meet these we will need to navigate the cryptic – often delicate questions of engagement and encounter: whether to? what? when? how? who? We can call all this 'vernacular psychology': an unschooled ancestor of current spawnings of systematic, academically-shepherded, formally packaged 'Clinical Psychology' and 'Psychological Treatments', with which most healthcare workers are now inculcated. Such vernacular psychology is guided by a quest for personal understanding, rather than any kind of 'objective' designation. Such understanding proceeds by asking questions: What is it like to be this other person, to have lived their life? What is the meaning and significance, for them, of this distress? What is the meaning and significance, for them, of me, now? What needs do I need to address that they might not (yet) be able to articulate?

---

[2] Zigmond, D (1987) *'Three types of encounter in the healing arts: dialogue, dialectic and didacticism'*. Holistic Medicine, Vol 2, 69-81

The language of such non-specialist forms of understanding can only succeed when fresh and personally meaningful. Unlike designatory language it can only be effective when our intelligence is fuelled and directed by resonance and imagination.[2] Procedural and technical language are, thus, often intrusive and antithetical to the vernacular; for languages not only communicates thought, it controls it. Vernacular psychology, with freedom of language and metaphor, seeks understanding before and beyond the shackles of our more administrative systems. When apposite it is a powerful element in the art of medicine and psychiatry. This is particularly well-illustrated in our best responses to those disabled by anguished dilemmas and unstable situations: the victims of life's shakings and tearings – the bereaved, the ravaged, the dispirited, the overwhelmed, the dying, the acutely mentally ill. These sufferers are different from those with stable and habitual patterns of distress: for such stability of distress is more likely to be receptive to our stability of approach – our reassuring and familiar structures: treatment planning, regular sessions, good-enough statistics, a premeditated and pre-packaged therapy, and so forth.

Across the wide span of palliative and curative activities, it is often vernacular psychology that best guides the kinds of empathic, compassionate approach that may enable containment and healing in the other. Being unschooled, it can be learned, by experience and apprenticeship, but probably not taught schematically: it is more the product of self-propelled education, rather than institutional training. This poses difficult conundrae for planners, managers and academics: it is easier to provide managed instruction than nurture nuances of culture.

It is worth reflecting on how important and widespread is our need for skilled, but unsystematised, psychology in our care of others. It is necessary even with the unconscious in ICU.

Shockingly, they are often much more conscious than we can bear, and they will remember.

There are many kinds of sufferers who are too dislocated and disintegrated by their distress to be able to attend to, or retain, our professionally systematised, management-modulated approaches: our 'Treatments'. They are, however, deeply influenced by sensible, sensitive understanding: communication that is bespoke, empathic, and prepared from fresh ingredients. These fresh ingredients are prepared to meet the (often) unarticulated and primitive needs of the sufferer. Rawly anguished, we all are likely to need some composite form of these: for validation, containment, comfort, encouragement, recognition, expression, understanding, catharsis or touch.[3][4] In such encounters, each matched cluster of responses will never be exactly repeated. These intimate choreographies are thus not susceptible to standardisation or measurement; they cannot be quantitatively researched, or mass-managed. Policy-makers, managers, eventually clinicians in the current quantification-centred culture, may become expediently neglectful, then oblivious.

With high levels of chaos or distress, the acutely mentally ill are usually unreceptive, or even obstructive, to our conveniently pre-packed, management-purchased, NICE-endorsed Shibboleth Therapies (CBT and MBT were cited in the article). Aspects of any of these *may* be helpful, but only if evoked as part of a developing dialogue. Not if we administer them, as a bolus, a prescribed procedure. A maze of semiotics here awaits us, for the extremely anguished are often beyond words: our dialogue has to be finely-tuned and respectfully empirical with the implicit. To enter this ever-evanescent realm

---

[3] Frank, J (1972) *Persuasion and Healing*. New York: Shocken

[4] Zigmond, D (Sept. 2010) *'Why would anyone use an unproven therapy? Treasures in the mist'*. Journal of Holistic Healthcare. Vol 7. Issue 2 17-19

of healing art we must be prepared to be delicate with ambiguity, improvisatory with our choreography: an exquisite and disciplined eclecticism. These, in turn, must aspire to an imaginatively accurate sense of what kind of explanations, language, metaphors and dialogue the sufferer is receptive to, and can bear. Such comprises much of healing, but how do we subsume it to 'Treatment'?

To end this article we should return to the beginning, to its title and that of the article that encouraged this enquiry. Can we best encounter the acutely mentally distressed by further administrative subdivisions, by further specialisms? What happens to holism, to sense and sensibility?

Clinical psychologists are no more qualified to enter this fragile and feral fray than any other clinicians. Frustratingly and fascinatingly, this is an area of marshland where our tarmacked roads quickly sink: we must find lighter ways to traverse. Psychologists can certainly contribute to these lighter ways; they can offer their slant of analytical thinking to protean processes. Our success usually depends upon our awareness and responsiveness to the vicissitudes of human complexity and paradox. This is a difficult and different stratum of activity and thought to that executised by the prescribed, planned and packaged.

We must beware, for the discounting of vernacular psychology, then its dismemberment, then colonisation by specialities, risks impoverishing or displacing the common compassion and emotional intelligence of us all.

Tennessee Williams starkly captures what so often eludes our over-organised and presumptuous encounters with others:

'I don't ask for your pity, but just your understanding – not even that, no – just your recognition of me in you, and the enemy, time, in us all.'

Tennessee Williams, *Sweet Bird of Youth* (1959)

Ω

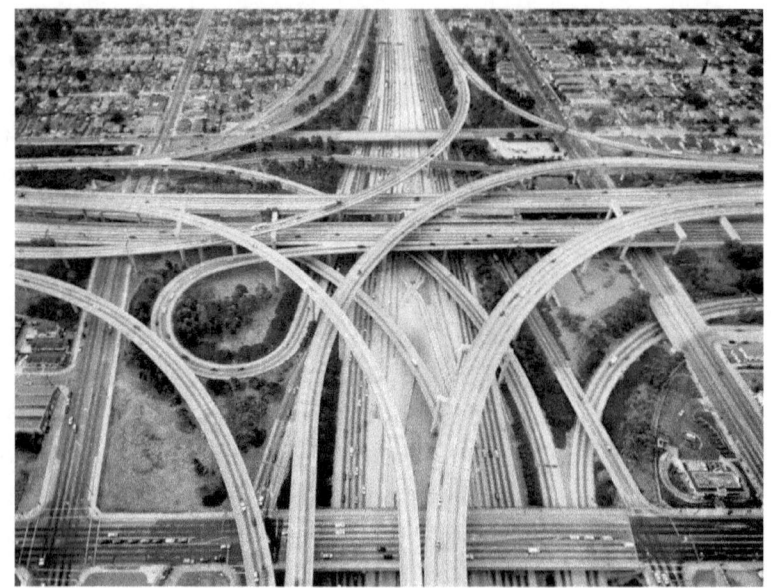

How to help Harry

Friend or Foe?
The scientific and the scientistic
in the fog of the frontline

Standardisation of medical services – increasingly by electronic monitoring, mediation and management – has become equated with 'best practice'. This seems to offer undeniable practical benefits: clarity, uniformity, reliability and ease of transmission. But does anything get lost? If so, what? how? why? This short exploration draws from authentic situations in Primary Care: a 'heartsink patient', and a problematic professional meeting. Usual conventions of disguise assure discretion.

We all want to be healthy. No one wants an unhealthy existence. And the job of Government is to help people live healthier lives.

Andrew Lansley MP, Secretary of State for Health, 23 January 2012

When you have duly arranged your 'facts' in logical order, lo, it is like an oil lamp that you have made, filled and trimmed, but which sheds no light unless you first light it.

Saint-Exupéry, *The Wisdom of the Sands* (1948)

Dr Q inhales Harry's fatalism involuntarily. It is not just the lingering and residual odours of his staple props – his tobacco and alcohol – but his anguish-laden physiology. This continues to signal Harry's troubles, both despite, and because of, his almost unceasing attempts to chemically banish, or at least quell, his morbidly echoing memories, his shame-leeched self-prophecies. Dr Q has come to surmise that such trapped and stultified internal worlds emanate particular kinds of energies and odours: that the physical experience becomes encoded, then signalled – in our sweat, our breath and in myriad thermal and electromagnetic transmissions we are usually unconscious of. He remembers an old designation connoting something similar: the 'heartsink patient'.

Dr Q has learned to be stoic and philosophical: he can look forward to enlivening counterpoint – very different people who energise the room with an aura of faith, trust and optimism. Reflecting on this, he now recalls conversations a couple of decades ago, when there was much talk of personal 'vibes': he never explored what scientific research has been done in this area, but his daily experience reminds him with recurring and fresh evidence of its power and centrality.

*

Harry's fatalism can be perceived more consciously, too: his trudging gait, the downcast gaze avoidant of the new or the personal, the sagging voice that has not the resolve to complete its message, his clothes and hair – clean enough – but habitually tousled, drab and dank.

Dr Q has known Harry fifteen years, and has witnessed and gleaned the story of Harry's cumulative desolation. In recent times Harry's already impoverished self-confidence was dealt a series of grievous blows: a marriage floundering from his difficulties of expression and extension, then foundering on their (his) infertility and poor employment prospects, then finally torpedoed by his wife's break-out: an affair with an 'old friend' – a confident, successful and expansive man whose attractiveness and fertility was soon evidenced by the pregnancy of Harry's future ex-wife.

In earlier times Harry conveyed to Dr Q descriptions and tales from his childhood. Of a father distant, fractious, discontent, hostile and critical. Of a mother softer, but lost in an ocean of melancholy. Her only child, she confided in him when he was old enough to 'understand'. Of the unhappy basis of her marital bond: the accidental conception of Harry in an untried relationship, ten years earlier. Of her attempts to conjure love through their Christian faith; through another conception soon after Harry – an obstetric disaster which cost mother her newborn, her womb and her future fertility.

Harry's childhood was spent trying to appease, comfort, compensate or placate those who gave him life. He could neither understand nor succeed.

Dr Q intuited something of this massive disseminated damage on their first encounter; later meetings confirmed and detailed. Dr Q's fuller portrait and biography of Harry grew slowly: piecemeal and opportunistically, for Dr Q was always careful not to encourage disclosure more than Harry could bear. Harry developed a reticent and shy trust: Dr Q sensed a flickering, bruised warmth.

Dr Q enlisted support. Psychiatrists at the times of Harry's greatest incapacity, counsellors when he could motivate himself a little more. Harry complied and they provided, at least, periodic containment for Harry and supportive respite for Dr Q. But Harry is a man of few words and little appetite for schematic enquiry: he did not respond to formal attempts at psychotherapy. His desolate view of himself and his world remains undiminished.

*

Harry does, however, entrust very limited aspects of himself to others. Now in his early middle-years, he has complied with his GP's practice screening programme. His blood lipids, checked for the first time, are found to be high. Dr Q remembers, too, Harry's response to the doctor's gentle enquiry regarding his feelings six months ago: Harry's father had just died suddenly of a heart attack. Harry had shrugged with a kind of glum defeat: 'he was never much of a father to me … now he's not here at all…'.

Dr Q was then mindful, not just of Harry's stunted grief, but of the portents, for Harry, for such a death. His emotional tangle of recent-upon-ancient frustrations and hurts, increasingly swallowed down with self-anaesthetising doses of booze, fags and factory foods augured badly. Now with father's sudden death these portents seemed clearer still: a sharpening prophecy.

The Practice receptionist's request for Harry to see Dr Q about his lipids was a standard procedure: 'to identify, discuss and take action regarding remediable risk factors'.

At the end of the last meeting, in the fresh shadow of his father's death, Dr Q had raised those specific concerns, again. The themes were old: the clarity was new. Harry responded with a rare vein of articulation, caustic and taut: 'I know your job is about saving lives, doctor, and I'm grateful for your kindness with me, but I'm not sure I have the kind of life that's worth saving … We can't all choose our lives and we've all got to die some time'. This quiet, courteous coda was undramatic in delivery, but arrestingly bleak in meaning. Dr Q had time only to express benign intent and tell Harry the bridge is always open.

*

Six months later, as the door opens, Dr Q knows it is Harry, booked in to discuss his lipids. These excess lipids may be the designated problem, but they represent the mere biochemical tip of a vast psycho-spiritual iceberg.

Dr Q holds his breath momentarily; he braces himself as he thinks: 'How to help Harry?'.

*

Stella has many similar meetings to address: her working days and diary are full. She has a friendly but business-like, diplomatic manner. This is reflected in her attire: trim knee-length navy skirt, cream blouse, discrete pearl earrings – a kind of uniform, smart but not alluring. Dr Q notices she is wearing her NHS Trust ID card around her neck, an emblem not just of how busy she is, but who controls her. This is a managed excursion.

Stella, though not herself medically trained, is the emissary of an expert group concerned with reducing cardiovascular disease. This committee has devised strategies and procedures which will be enacted by all relevant health practitioners. Stella's job is to brief and instruct the practitioners: to assure professional compliance for The Plan. Such compliance relieves practitioners of individual judgement and discrimination: The Plan prescribes and directs. Invisible experts decide.

Dr Q is sitting amidst his peers, local GPs. Stella is explaining the latest addition to The Plan. A new computer program is being introduced. The practitioners will feed in the relevant clinical data, and the computer will calculate the statistical chance of morbidity and mortality. This 'scientific' prediction is then shared with the patient for discussion and action. The GPs will receive an extra payment for compliance: Dr Q notices the galvanising ripple of interest and attention.

Dr Q recently attended his own GP and received the kind of consultation that The Plan spawns. Dr Y was young, brisk, authoritative. Her attention was rapt to the computer screen, where she quickly garnered and collated abstracted data. The computer prophesised favourably for Dr Q's fate. Dr Y spoke for The Oracle, as she turned from the computer screen towards him: 'That's not too bad, not too bad at all…'. She illustrated her prognostic cheeriness with some itemised statistics. Her smile seemed winsome, but Dr Q wondered who the smile was for: he was doubtful how much she had really perceived him. There had been little real discussion. Beyond medical questions, she enquired little. Dr Q did not introduce himself as a fellow-GP: his curiosity was then roused, to see what a 'standard' consultation was like. Was the smile another impersonal, though decorative, generic procedure? What is a smile to someone unseen?

Dr Q is thinking about Stella's financially-enhanced instructions, his own experience with Dr Y and how these would be templated with Harry. As he understands this, he is being paid to prime the computer, which then primes him to then say to Harry something like: 'Harry, we have fed all your available personal and family health and lifestyle data into the computer program. Your computed five-year risk for combined cardio/cerebrovascular events is 38.73%. This comprises a 14.71% mortality group, leaving another 24.02% with significant morbidity events. For your age group, this is very high risk … We can provide you with category subgroup differential analyses, if you wish …'

Dr Q is wondering how such formulaic and statisticised thinking or communication can possibly further help Harry, or many others that Dr Q sees. Dr Q's monitoring and conversations, for many years, have approached the complex issues of self-protection and self-care, but in a form and language that are personal and vernacular – not those predicated by the technical: tethered to the computer, or decided by distant expert committees.

Dr Q puts such notions to Stella. He adds that he has long-regarded what, when and how to share with each person, in each situation, as a delicate, complex but fundamental skill in Medical Practice. A good example of what anchors holistic medicine as an interpersonal art, a humanity.

Stella listens politely, nodding periodically, looking tired. Dr Q imagines her nodding represents fatigued diplomacy, rather than engaged understanding.

She reiterates how the computer program has been designed by a team of experts, and it behoves us to follow their lead. In addition, conveying quantitative information to patients, in a way that can itself be quantified, confers clear advantages to the management of practitioners, in their management of patients. 'I think you'll agree, doctor, it will make your treatment of these patients more *scientific*, and that has to be good for all of us…'

Dr Q thinks Stella is proposing this – especially her emphasised word 'scientific' – as an ineluctable summary. But Dr Q has many doubts and caveats. How to engage and interest another person in changing deeply established psychological patterns regarding their relationship to themselves, their body and their fate is often not a simple matter of data, formulation and instruction. Such complexity requires thoughtful investment in interpersonal interest, contact and understanding: activities far less accessible to quantification and science. Will not The Plan eclipse these subtle but important endeavours?

Yet Stella's declamation on the uncontentious blessings of anything that appears scientific represents a wider, currently thriving, kind of hypnotic rhetoric – a cultural ideology. The presentation of an apparent vocabulary and syntax of science becomes more important than its meaning for the participants.

Appearing scientific becomes an end in itself, a new kind of Shibboleth. Science as a posture, a garment, a cultural or status commodity becomes *scientism*.

Dr Q attempts to courteously and concisely condense this for Stella, but she is now more restive than receptive.

'Look', she says, 'you don't have to think about all that, because you'll be paid for it': a tired teacher attempting to control the end of a difficult class.

Another doctor, Dr S, turns to Dr Q, looks at his watch impatiently and offers Stella tetchy support: 'Yes, I can't see what all this is about. What won't you understand?! You're getting paid for it!'

Dr Q thinks he does understand, very well. But he remembers different kinds of meetings, twenty years ago, where they had very different kinds of discourse. He found these much more valuable. He would like to talk with them now about how to help Harry.

Ω

Information is pretty thin stuff, unless mixed with experience.

Clarence Day, *The Crow's Nest* (1921)

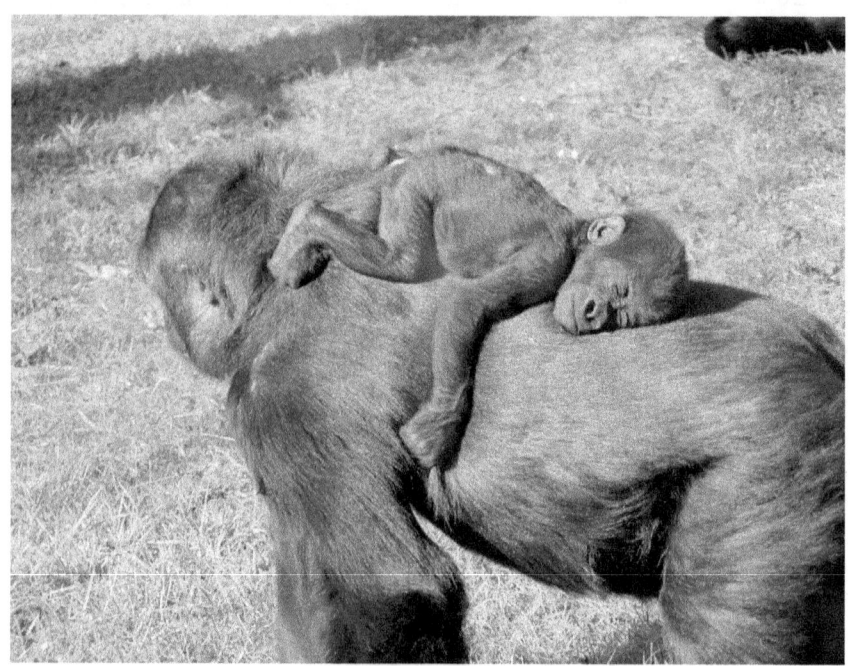

Eric

*- diagnosis may be sometimes necessary;
it is rarely sufficient*

Diagnostically centred, schematic and managed healthcare has brought great benefit to the treatment of structural physical diseases. With other kinds of dis-ease its results are often much more problematic, even destructive. Current trends render this a growing problem. A true and recent story of an eternally grief-stricken elderly man serves as a cautionary and explanatory example.

Introduction

Diagnoses – when well placed – have muscular leverage: they form the core-knowledge of most of our dramatically successful treatments for structural physical illnesses. Yet diagnoses have limitations of view; they can only offer descriptive clusters of commonality – what is generally true, the generic. They cannot tell us about the unique world of *this* individual *now*.

For this reason the generic diagnosis often fares poorly in healthcare realms where individual understanding, meaning and experience hold the key to therapeutic engagement. It is proposed here that most psychiatry, therapeutic psychology and medical encounters with functional complaints are all better addressed by a more idiomorphic approach; that the cost of not doing so is high.

Why is this important? What can happen? The following true story, about Eric, explains and illustrates.

This account is an extract from a long letter to a Director of a Mental Health Trust. The letter is written to document, and then catalyse, thought and debate about the increasingly inordinate use of the medical model – how this is leading to a complex fragmentation, and then destructive depersonalisation, of healthcare. Alarmingly this is happening especially in areas where quality and continuity of human contact and individual understanding is most important.

The story of Eric, and its inherent missed and miscommunications are a small but powerful example of a grave and accelerating problem. The letter could have been written to any similar NHS Trust. The discerned problems are now so widespread and insidious as to best be considered cultural.

The wide and complex sources of this culture are beyond the scope of this article. Yet we can begin a remedial response. Any limitation or reversal of damage must come from a counter-cultural ethos: I call this 'holistic compassionate care' (HCC). Some essential and guiding features of HCC are itemised in the box below.

Holistic, compassionate care: a summary

- Personal healthcare is a humanity guided by science.
- This humanity is an ethos and an art.
- Holistic, compassionate care (HCC) requires mindful titration of art and science in ever-changing situations.
- This titration works like a carburettor: balancing opposing elements (petrol:science v air:art) in ever-changing mixtures to serve the needs of the whole (engine:person).
- Too much or too little of any one element causes suboptimal functioning and, eventually, no function at all.
- HCC is potentially important in all our encounters with human distress or dysfunction, yet always differently.
- HCC is particularly important in situations where there is not a quick and decisive physical treatment – hence General Practice, Psychology and Psychiatry are especially vulnerable to its loss.
- HCC often deals with issues that are personal, inexplicit and have symbolic meaning. Science has no access to such 'metacommunication'.
- HCC is often potent, but subtle and fragile. It is easily damaged or destroyed. Its 'habitat' needs protection.
- HCC is currently seriously damaged and impaired by an excess of 'science' and corresponding impoverishment of 'art'. [This is much like the carburettor delivering a 'too rich' mixture: the engine will have difficulties with fuel consumption, environmental pollution, power, smooth-running and starting. Healthcare analogies are obvious.]
- Thus more of something 'good' may, in fact, be worse.
- Schematisation is the opposing principle to holism. Thus, for example, excessive category-based management will

displace attachment-based personal understanding. Examples of current changes adding to this inadvertent damage: in General Practice – the loss of smaller, friendlier practices and personal lists for GPs, QOF-based remuneration; in Psychiatry – increasing subdivisions of medically-modelled care pathways and Clinical-Academic Groups; in Psychology – very similar: especially in excessive, diagnostically schematised CBT/IAPTS pathways.

- Wisdom = knowledge x reflection x experience x imagination.
- Systems that replace clinical wisdom with managerial solidarity generate very serious problems.

'It is easier to know (and understand) men in general than one man in particular.'

La Rochefoucauld, *Maxims* (1665)

1977-2010

As a GP for more than thirty years in the same practice, I have had medical responsibility for thousands of people. Eric was one of my few 'old-timers' I'd had almost no contact with. I knew what he looked like: a tall, increasingly stooped, bespectacled man, now in his early 70s, who had always dressed with neat, quiet formality and who carried a mien of discrete compliance, of well-mannered appeasement. I remembered several glimpses – spread over many years – of his visits to other practitioners. Paradoxically, I had another route of acquaintance with him that was more detailed – though more abstract – through the post: letters from specialists over many decades. Hazy memories of these were crystallised into the terminology of his disease-register and medical notes summary: 'Mature-onset Diabetes' and a 'long history of major, relapsing depression'. I remembered old letters from the 1960s: the days of outer-city Mental Hospitals, 'modern' tricyclic antidepressants and courses of ECT. More recent letters had better news: containment and quiescence of his symptoms and punctilious compliance with prescriptions, plans and attendance. I sensed stable fragility well attended to: I had no need to intervene or understand further: if at peace, do not disturb.

*

2011-2012

An urgent phone call. The receptionist, Sue, correctly recognises raw and intelligent fear in the unknown woman's voice. Sue is intelligent, in response. It is not a 'good time' for phone calls, but she puts the call through immediately. Sue has an unschooled instinct for real distress, and thus accurate precedence.

'Doctor, I'm Dora, Eric's niece ... I've known him all my life ... I've never seen him as bad as this, so 'down' ... since last week I can't get him to eat, or talk, or take care of himself ... I can't really get normal conversation from him ... he's said frightening things: all quiet and intense – about his life ending, or ending his life – I can't really tell ... I can't leave him like this, but I live out of London and have young children to get back to ... I don't know what do, doctor, can you help? ...'

*

Within an hour, Eric and Dora are sitting with me. Eric's deflation, hopelessness and anguish are painfully and immediately apparent: his slow movement, enfeebled voice, depleted gaze and burdened gait all convey intense and incarcerated despair. Words – delicately baited – may later amplify or explain. Dora's presence and prescience are what I had imagined from our brief telephone contact: unintrusively engaged, lovingly watchful, fearful of tragic catastrophe.

I sense in Eric some fresh personal trauma causing this dramatic collapse: some kind of rupture; an internal haemorrhage of hope and faith. I need his words to explain: they are like frightened small fish sheltering in the darkened deep. I have to be still awhile, and patient. His words begin to surface; I lean forward, gently, to catch them:

'They've told Nancy that I can't see her anymore, that I've got to go somewhere else … but I don't want to go somewhere else … I just want to go back to see Nancy …'

The words almost collapse at the back of his throat and are exhaled plaintively and weakly, as if he is dying. They choke to a halt with inhaled, silent sobs.

Dora is calmer, now she is sharing this enervated burden. I turn to look at her. She returns a knowing gaze. She does: she starts to explain:

'Uncle Eric has been seeing Nancy (a Social Worker) at the Clifton (Community Mental Health Centre) for about eight years. He's been told he has to stop. Nancy says it's due to some sort of reorganisation: that the Managers have told Nancy that what she's doing isn't what's most suitable for him: that they'll find him somewhere else … But I know how much my uncle has been helped by Nancy: he only sees her for about twenty minutes, every few weeks. But he trusts her, and she's been kind and really got to understand him over a long time. I think that's why he's been so well for these last years … After everything that happened to him when he was young, taking Nancy away from him now seems so cruel …'

I realise I am dealing with broken vital connections, and a still-active volcanic personal ancient history, of which I know nothing. I must understand the essence of Eric's world, and story, very quickly.

Within fifteen minutes I have deciphered much: I am simultaneously gratified by understanding and disturbed by what I have understood.

*

Eric was the youngest of five boys in a traditional, poor London docker's family. His mother, in her forties when he was born, ailed throughout Eric's infancy and died when he was three. He was cared for by a younger sister of his dead mother, Aunt Ada, until the onset of the Blitz. By the time his neighbourhood was shattered and ablaze, he and his four brothers and father had all dispersed, separately, away from London: Eric and three brothers were evacuated to families throughout the Home Counties, the oldest brother and father joined the Merchant Navy, hoping to stay together. They did not; father perished in an attack on the Arctic Convoy.

Eric's wartime childhood as an evacuee was abject, grief-struck and fearful. He was moved several times to different families for reasons dictated to him, but little understood by him. His experiences of care were various – kindness, affection, hostility, cruelty, indifference – but never predictable, dependable or within his control. He could not understand the difference between death, separation, abandonment or punishment. He learned to survive by appeasement, submission, invisibility. His memories of his mother and Aunt Ada brought grief that was rarely consoled: he learned, too, to appear to be brave.

At the end of The War, at the age of eleven, he returned to his orphaned family of older brothers, in the resuscitated ruins of London's Docklands. Eric's brothers were kindly and protective with Eric, though tougher than he: they had had long-enough and robust mothering. For his sense of protection and belonging, he followed his Band of Brothers to work in the Docks, soon after leaving school.

Eric's brothers and a few of his more thoughtful workmates were his social and family life, for several decades: he never made sexual relationships with women – a dangerous and painful yearning, a Bridge Too Far.

Eric's depressive breakdowns, in his thirties and forties, were possibly related to fresh abandonments: by his brothers who left him, each to move away from the Docklands to spawn their own families. By his fifties his 'family' consisted of his now distant, elderly, often ailing, brothers and a few retiring, soon-to-vanish, fellow dockers.

As his livelihood, companionship and brothers died, this vulnerable, inarticulately yearning, self-deprecating elderly man feared the waning of his solitary life, unknown and unwitnessed. Nancy had recognised this with discrete intuition, and for several years provided the kind of family surrogacy that provides humble but deep affiliation and palliation, yet has no official designation. Nancy, it seems, was guided by a basic tenet of care: that to be known to another, with intimacy and volition, is one of the most powerful balms for human distress. With evident sense and sensitivity Nancy had – with necessary professional safeguards and boundaries – contained and symbolically cradled this eternally grieving, unmothered old man. Nancy's humbly potent humanity, though, had invidious flaws: it is undesignated and unmeasurable; not part of a recognised generic care pathway. Ipso facto, Nancy should not be doing this work: Eric should go elsewhere, to a place of prescribed and recognised 'treatments'.

The consequences of this 'rationalised management'? An avoidably, yet now primitively disturbed and distressed elderly man – whose life I now fear for. What will I do?

*

What I can. My attentions to, and on behalf of, Eric have been multifarious, and for many months. My more direct endeavours have been akin, I imagine, to Nancy's – to compassionately contain, respond and guide: to comfort, palliate and help him reclaim some hope for his increasingly meagre life. Due to his feelings of unsafety now, with the Mental Health Teams, I have been seeing him every two weeks:

I accept I may need to do this indefinitely. I am sadly aware that there are now few GPs who would take this initiative, or accept this responsibility. What would happen to Eric elsewhere?

I have directed my attention more widely, too. I have wanted to understand and define the institutional misperceptions and misconceptions: how, with apparent good intent, do we deliver such miscarriages and perversions of care? I have had to be resilient and assiduous in my (re)search, motivated not only by Eric's individual and affecting predicament, but also an increasing number of other patients describing similar dislocations of human understanding by Specialist Services.

Over many months I have made numerous phone calls to various Psychiatric Teams. I have had to be patient, persistent and assertive to generate substantial dialogue. Face-to-face contact has been harder, success had been sporadic yet labour-intensive.

This Odyssey has two parallel paths – of seeking exploratory dialogue with Psychiatric Services while securing restitution of care for Eric. Both are long and difficult. This following description thus attempts salience, not completeness.

*

I spoke initially to Nancy, then to both the Clinical Manager and the Consultant Psychiatrist at the Mental Health Team. With all three there was a layered carapace to their responses. First, wary bewilderment: why would a GP want to enter their territory with such energy of concern and enquiry? Then institutional deflection and edict: 'The Team has assessed and decided ...'. 'The Care Pathway, directed by agreed Trust Protocol ...' and other armoured phrases of unpeopled authority. With skill and patience I was able to get to the cramped and uncomfortable person trapped behind the armour.

Nancy seemed wary, weary, circumspect then relieved in her brief confiding:

'I'm sorry, Doctor ... of course, I'm especially sorry that poor Eric is having to go through any of this ... I'm sorry that I can't do the helpful work I know and like ... I'm sorry you're having to deal with the fall-out of all this ... But I can't do anything – you know how it is with Management these days: I can't say too much ...'

The others, with less direct knowledge of Eric, went through the same process of deflection, dissemblance, then confident and dispirited contrition.

Again, my tricky choreographic riddle: how to maintain respectful colleaguial relationships, while indicating clearly and strongly my wide-ranging disagreements with their policies and decisions?

My clarity and resolve – and anxious concern – were refuelled unhappily; by the accuracy of my predictions: Eric's abject misery became so uncontained that he was admitted to a Psychiatric Unit. Given his early experiences of care by strangers and the nature of current admission centres, his likely reaction was also easily predicted: iatrogenic damage was deepened. The cost to NHS resources is considerable; to human welfare much greater.

*

In my effort to keep Eric's distress closer to drama than tragedy, I contacted you in your role of Clinical Director for the Mental Health Trust. Your response was prompt, concerned and pragmatic: you delegated one of your experienced and Senior Deputies, Dr Y, who would communicate with me.

Dr Y did contact me in a way that was remarkably unremarkable: he sent me a long e-mail.

Remarkable? Unremarkable? Which?

The e-mail combines immediacy and precision of signal with remoteness of human contact: no face, no voice, no location, no touch. Yet it is increasingly used automatically, even in such humanly-demanding situations; it has become a part of our culture. But is such signalling communication? If so, what kind? What for?

Dr Y's e-mail was polite in taking control. It proceeded like an Instruction Manual, assuming that I needed his executive explanation, guidance and help. Some anomalies made this most improbable. He started by acknowledging that his reply was mostly based on his perusal of electronic records: he had never met Eric, 'but I do have a lot of experience with such patients'. As if I do not?

Proceeding to address me like a silent tannoy system, Dr Y then raised the possible therapeutic options of various psychotherapies for Eric. This line of thought seemed (to me) to assume a common simplistic notion of 'psychotherapy' as a sequestered, distilled, specialist activity that has to be designated and delivered systematically. Eric (and I would say most people I see who are distressed) do not want or need that kind of schematised activity. They do, however, want contacts that are psychotherapeutic: contacts that develop trust, hope, understanding, meaning, structure and safety. Nancy had been doing this with Eric, very appositely, for years. I could see this clearly within minutes of talking to Eric. Even Sue, my receptionist, rapidly intuited much the same. Yet various managers of Specialist Services could not, or would not allow themselves, to see this. Why? My theory: because Nancy's unschooled and undesignated therapeutic contact lay outside currently prescribed algorithms and care pathways: that which is not prescribed now becomes proscribed.

Dr Y's long and tendentious e-mail concluded, with a kind of magisterial authority, by instructing me about this man he had never met: 'Overall, the type of all-embracing care that secondary care tends to offer can often entrench such personality characteristics'. What does this mean? Like most general statements about human experience, motivation or Fate, this is a notion that is bound to be true, sometimes. But an opposite proposition is also sometimes true. The art and wisdom of practice comes from the creative and pragmatic editing and synthesis of such partial truths. So, Dr Y's statement, which may sometimes be usefully true, is now rendered hazardous by its introduction as 'Overall', which implies hegemony, like a monarch reigning 'over all'. This is not pedantry: a crucial and difficult part of our work in Mental Health is to always look for exceptions to our predicated patterns. Without skilful handling of these paradoxes, important misunderstandings will be frequent. Eric is a stark example of this, and how it happens. Dr Y's long and didactic e-mail seemed heedless of this. He paid no attention to the personal nature of Eric or my engagement with him: Eric will need some kind of innominate, but bespoke, humanely imaginative containment until the end of his life. This is not rare, yet is rarely acknowledged. Over many years of working with the mentally distressed, I see that this kind of innominate approach has been crucial. How do we assure space and resources for such unpackaged, difficult-to-measure-yet-made-to-measure, free-form compassionate contact with others? In the longer term, in contrast, I have found the currently vaunted time-limited, designated packages of care to be of evanescent interest and shallow effect.

What I wanted and needed from Dr Y was some sophistication of dialogue. What I got was a default-type of e-mail: now so ubiquitous as to be a new convention. In this culture – of screen-before-person – practitioners are now deluged by an inassimilable quantity of such signals. Few get read with good attention; even fewer intelligently discussed. Yet, if we look closely, we can see anomalies and absurdities which few would intend. This happened here: with Dr Y, myself and Eric.

*

Let us distance ourselves and look with an alien, intelligent eye. What do we see? In a highly complex arena of mental distress, where individual understanding must be key to any success, a delegated manager electronically transmits abstracted judgements and decisions. He has spoken neither to the patient nor to either of the most involved practitioners, both of whom are highly experienced, competent and intelligent. He is addressing one of them now, but does not draw on their knowledge and experience of their work or the patient. His view is, rather, distilled from absent persons' computerised records, and then submitted to 'authoritative' patterns of generic recommendations (to which there must always be many exceptions). The role of this sequestered manager is not to engage in a mutually informative dialogue with those involved. Instead, he 'posts' a long, monologous electronic signal, with intent to instruct and command. A related image occurs to me: of an Air Traffic Officer in a control tower. He is looking into a screen at symbolic representations of distant aircraft, to which he sends vectoring instructions. I have little doubt that this may be the best format for Air Traffic Control. But electronically mediated remote control for mentally distressed humans? What kind of psychiatry does this lead to?

We have here sampled what is coming.

For many years I worked in and alongside Mental Health Services where such formulaic management hardly existed, but intelligent collegial personal contact was abundant, welcome, even enjoyed. In all the places I worked, until recently, I witnessed the likes of Eric receiving flexible and humane care: schematic designation might have been comparatively meagre, but the human understanding and its quiet satisfactions much greater.

*

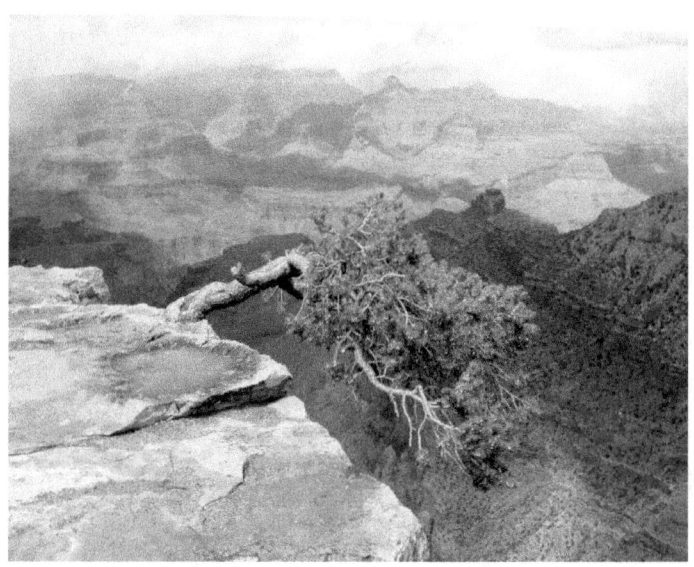

I have been striving to reconnect with – maybe even begin to regenerate – this older, more humanly-earthed professional culture. Due to my frustrations with this I contact you. But due to your business (I imagine) you delegate my request for dialogue to a trusted lieutenant, Dr Y. He, quite unintentionally (I believe) then rapidly re-enacts the bulk of my problems and discontent with NHS Institutions: he resorts to a device which short-circuits any personal contact, understanding or complexity: without further ado he transmits a didactic e-mail, defining reality to me, and for me. I don't mind this approach if I am enquiring about train times, but I want to talk about Eric. I am reminded of a Woody Allen aphorism: 'Confidence is what you have before you have understood the problem'.

Dr Y's rapid acting-out of my critique amused me as an exquisitely timed though inadvertent parody; but it simultaneously dismayed me with further evidence of the ubiquity of the problem. Yet I have hope. Firstly, that you have read this long-journeyed and thought-marinated marathon letter with good attention. Then, most importantly, I hope that dialogue will be broadened and deepened, between us and beyond us. Lastly, I hope you do not answer this with a formulaic e-mail!

Ω

'It is the critical vision alone which can mitigate the unimpeded operation of the automatic.'

Marshall Mcluhan, *The Mechanical Bride* (1951)

Publ. in *Journal of Holisti Healthcare Vol 9 Iss. 2 2012*

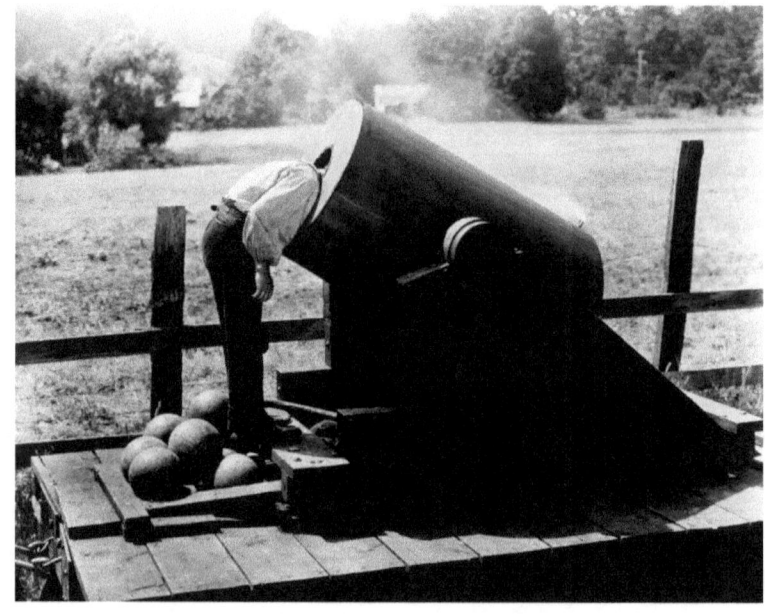

Buster Keaton *The General* 1926

Fallacies in Blunderland

Overschematic overmanagement:
perverse healthcare

Introduction

For more than twenty years there have been various devices to create an internal market central to the NHS: Fiefdom-like Trusts, commercial-type commissioning, contractually defined 'purchasers' and 'providers' of healthcare are current examples. The resulting commodification and commercialisation of healthcare has become its own culture. What does all this look like at the frontline? The following authentic vignettes from contemporary General Practice provide a view. Only usual devices of disguise subtract from accuracy.

The first two tales are now commonplace and superficially trivial, but they already contain the possibilities of bureaucratic burden and distortion that make the shocking last two stories more understandable.

*

'It is a bad plan that admits of no modification.'

Pubilius Syrus, *Moral Sayings* (1st century BC)

'Tis not the habit that maketh the monk.'

Thomas Fuller, *Gnomolgia* (1732)

*

1. Trivial tales: serious themes

A. The Loop

Dr T receives a letter from Mr O, an orthopaedic consultant. It is about Sheila, a healthy spirited woman of 40 who sustained a severe and displaced fracture of both bones of one ankle. She required surgery to realign the distorted bones, then plates and screws to secure them. All of this has gone well, but several weeks later her ankle remains painfully stiff. Sheila will need physiotherapy. Will Dr T please refer her?

This is not as innocent or straightforward as it may seem. A historical explanation:

Several years ago, before the fragmentation of our national service into parochial Trusts, such collateral work was usually done with speed, accuracy, ease, friendliness and very little, but essential and useful, documentation. Mr O would have spoken to his well-known Clinic Physiotherapist, Carol, and said, in effect: 'Carol, this is Sheila (and her problem) that you can help by doing "X". Let me know if there's any unusual difficulty. I'll see her again in six weeks'. Dr T may have been informed, but not involved.

Recent times and ideologies have moved to more complex procedures. Trusts now mistrustfully contend and vie, sell and buy. Mr O now has no such sensible and 'homely' arrangement with his physiotherapist (or anyone else). The commissioning health-economy mandates that fragmentation of services is introduced to generate extra revenue for his Trust. Thus Physiotherapy is now separately tariffed from Fracture Orthopaedics. Mr O must now write to Sheila's GP, Dr T, suggesting that Sheila be referred back to the hospital for Physiotherapy. Although Mr O is far better placed than Dr T to make this decision and to implement it, the new commissioning system disincentivises this. This is because the interposed administrative loop 'earns revenue' for his Trust, by 'selling' necessary physiotherapy services. This added complexity helps ensure the financial viability of the fiefdoms.

What does this mean? A short link is turned into a long loop: it is not just Dr T's professional time and attention that are distracted by this unproductive artifice – this must now involve clerks, IT coders, contract administrators, accountants, auditors. Such long threads lead to tangles, so Personnel and Contract Managers and Lawyers must be added.

The aggrandisement snowballs: physiotherapy must now present as more arcane and formidable. Mr O cannot simply make a collegial (if highly competent) request: such must be replaced by detailed referral forms, team referral meetings, documented referral thresholds and criteria, data collection and collation (however specious), the propagation of professional reports that illusion depth through length, and gravitas through the unnecessary elaboration of technical language.

Such seriousness must be suitably framed: Carol cannot simply and quickly decide – from her considerable experience – what to offer Sheila. Sheila must join a waiting list for a long, over-inclusive, formulaic assessment to be performed. This will be documented in assiduous and trivial detail, then sent to Dr T, though Dr T has no interest or use for this. He certainly has not asked for it. However, for the 'providers' of physiotherapy it bestows auras of completeness and complexity: devices of theatrical rhetoric and justification. A new, and now necessary, language of survival: Lebensraum.

Dr T has become an increasing though unwilling recipient of such over-laden and other-agendad communications. He now receives hundreds of e-mails every week whose purpose is not to communicate with him about what he needs to know and what may interest him, but rather to confer some kind of aura of immunity, impunity or importance around the sender.

Dr T, despite many years of diligent, competent practice, remains anxiously conscientious: he reads such letters, warding off an attrition of fatigued alienation and ... resentment. He hankers for a previous era of more straightforward communications from colleagues who wrote pragmatically of what he wanted or needed to know: a culture where help came from personal connections, not a kind of commercialised totalitarianism. He sighs with unsentimental sadness and sagged purpose. He imagines restitution in early retirement.

B. Size 13 Moonboot

Mustafa is an athletic young man, very tall and with large feet. While playing in a football away-match he fractures a metatarsal bone in his foot. He is seen by the accident doctor at the home counties hospital (HCH) who says to him: 'It's a straightforward minor fracture: your body will slowly heal it, but you'll need a Moonboot for several weeks to get around. You've got very large feet: unfortunately we don't have any size 13 in stock. But you live close to the large London hospital (LLH): they are bound to have some. Just go along to their accident department and they will fit you up. It will be quite straightforward ...'

That was true until recent years. It is now very different.

Mustafa goes to the accident department of LLH. After a long wait he is curtly told that as this is not a fresh injury he will need a referral from his GP, Dr T. Mustafa sees Dr T, tired at the end of a morning infiltrated and obstructed by such bureaucratic formalities and ritualistic documentation. Dr T writes a clear request for the Moonboot and a routine follow up, with an equally clear and concise account of the background problem. Until the recent past this would have been responded to in kind.

Not now.

Mustafa reattends LLH accident department with Dr T's letter. A triage nurse peruses it briefly before consulting a Manager. She returns to deliver an accurate slow-spinner: Dr T is bowled-out with her first ball: 'Your doctor and HCH obviously don't understand the system. We can't just give you a Moonboot. You have to be formally referred to Orthopaedics, and then a proper assessment has to be made by a Specialist...'

Dr T had not really understood the concepts of a 'purchaser/provider split', 'Commissioning' and related notions to focus and facilitate healthcare. He is learning now as Mustafa's agent, in these shuttlecock exchanges between Trusts: through these frustrations he is becoming familiar with the procedures, language and protocol.

What he has not learned – what he cannot see – is the value of all this to his patients, or his own efforts on their behalf. Amidst his many conversations – seeking to clarify the benefits of such systems – he talks with Dr Q.

2. Absurd but true: A corrupt cadenza
– how the schematic becomes perverse

Dr Q is, like Dr T, a stalwart member of an older but dwindling species: a single-handed, vocationally-motivated, psychologically-minded family doctor. He is a quiet man of understated but sustained and sustaining warmth and laconic humour. Professionally close, in both geography and ethos, Drs Q and T meet for companionable support, ventilation and experienced guidance. Dr Q listens, and identifies with bemused and increasing frustration: he has experienced his own varieties of The Loop and Moonboot.

'I've got one to appal and amuse you ... Yes, both! ... But I have to be careful who I tell ...' says Dr Q, teasing gently with competition and conspiracy.

He talks of one of the many institutional directives attempting to raise the standards of practitioners and practices. Most such devices are now measured, scored and complexly linked to remuneration. He is describing one yoked to substantial (written) complaints from patients. Each practice must now show evidence of how it responds to the complainant, and then turns this to positive reflection, learning and changes in their procedure and organisation.

Dr Q slowly unravels his tangle of frustrations: 'Of course, I agree with the better philosophy behind all this: listening, looking, thinking from another's viewpoint; not being too busy, proud or fragile to reflect on, or share such variations.

'So far, so good – but from here it gets worse, for me anyway. You see, I've spent a working lifetime really interested in these complexities. Probably because of that I haven't had any substantial complaint for about twenty years. That's an achievement I'm happy with, but the absurdity is that my practice has lost substantial income through being unable to complete the exercise. For the last few years I have been financially penalised because no one has complained about me!

'Well, my Practice Manager, Muriel, has many abilities but I hadn't realised how she is also a Mistress of Dark Arts. She quietly conjured a miniature masterpiece: she forged a fictitious letter of complaint; invented a practice meeting to respond to this with discussion, reflection and action plans; provided minutes of the (non) meeting, and a summary report for the monitoring authorities. The result of all this? We invent a complaint, because we don't have one, write a long bogus report for an authority that doesn't read it, and then claim the same money as everybody else! Is that a good way to spend doctors' time or NHS money?' Dr Q expresses his rhetorical coda: 'Righteous fraud!', he laughs sharply, a kind of self-parodic cymbal-clash.

But now a cross-current of doubt, more hesitant. He clears his throat: 'That's not the way I normally behave, is it? … I mean, what would you do?'

Dr T has not expected this earnest question. He shrugs self-consciously, while attempting awkwardly to combine expressions of fraternal collusion with innocent bewilderment. This is difficult: finding the right formula of words impossible. He shelters behind an enigmatic smile.

3. Absurd but tragic: When Care Pathways obliterate care

'I don't think I can do it any more, doctor. I think she needs to be looked after somewhere else ... I'm not as strong as I used to be ... I can't lift her, especially if she falls. And now she's much more confused and gets upset in ways that I can't reason with her about ... It's so hard, doctor: I think it might kill me ...'

Dr T thinks he is not exaggerating: it might. Cyril is aged nearly ninety, Iris is ninety-four. They married seventy years ago, a wartime marriage. As a twenty-year-old signaller with the Royal Navy protecting the Atlantic Convoys, his hunger to marry Iris had been talismanic as well as romantic: he somehow believed that ritualising the strength of his love would protect him, help him survive. He had, and forty years later he had described to a young Dr T his then-unspoken war-time terror, and the transcendent power of his faith-in-love.

Iris had been a very attractive younger woman, but ravaged by primitive anxieties: severe early losses and cruelties had been semi-healed by Cyril's loving devotion, but her wounds were shaken open by a late miscarriage. The subsequent birth of a son assuaged but did not resolve. Dr T remembers reading the unusually neat fountain-penned notes of his predecessor, referring to her 'numerous functional complaints' and her 'polymorphous anxiety'. From the 1980s Dr T would help guide Iris through this hazily mapped, apparently endless, medical wilderness. His patience and imagination were his most important resources, but Cyril was his most important ally. For more than thirty years Dr T witnessed the finest manifestations of loving devotion, *Agape*: indefatigable support, humorous affection, practical containment. Cyril was happy in his role of loving protector: Dr T was appreciated for his professional support and guidance. There followed a long period of eddied stability, until the onset of Iris's dementia.

*

As so often, the dementia was first signalled insidiously and ambiguously, in her ninetieth year. Unsighted by retinal degeneration and unwilling to wear her hearing aid, this frail and slight old lady became increasingly difficult to contact. Her confusion of place and persons was distressing. Her shards of insight even more so: with angrily tearful eruption she would rage at her humiliated disintegration: Cyril tended her with quiet, soft tears of sorrow.

When Cyril developed his increasingly untreatable heart failure he knew that his tide, too, was running out. 'I just want to be able to look after her long enough, doctor …' he had said with characteristic, stoic courtesy.

*

When Cyril – looking haggard, exhausted and afraid – talks with polite deference of his inability to cope and a premonition of his death, Dr T has no doubt about the need for urgent action. Iris needs immediate respite care. He calls Social Services.

*

Many years ago Dr T recalls a similarly abject and acutely disintegrating situation, and his similar request. He remembers his meeting and conversations with the Social Worker, Phyllis, a thoughtful, sensible middle-aged woman with maternal warmth and grand-maternal wisdom. Phyllis had been quick and seamless in her understanding and intelligent actions. Dr T had thought that such dextrous and humane holistic engagement had transformed a painfully tragic situation into one with a kind of elegant pathos. He had felt grateful, moved and proud to be associated with such unglamourised expertise.

*

Now, in 2012, it is very different. Dr T is phoning the duty-desk Social Worker, Vanessa. He is trying to convey, with intelligible rapidity, the nature of his problem with Iris and

Cyril: a brief history and his urgent recommendations. This is turning out to be very difficult. Vanessa clearly has another agenda. Her voice sounds young to Dr T. She transmits it with manicured, polite cautiousness. She explains a protocol which must be adhered to: preliminary screening questions must be completed. Existing Social Services' package? Home OT Assessment? Number of falls? Mental competence? Screening blood tests? Complete Medical and Psychiatric history? Most recent Social Services assessment? Yes, yes, yes ... and YES! Dr T attempts to tell Vanessa that a collegial dialogue can get to the important points more accurately and quickly. But Vanessa is well briefed and disciplined: she sticks to her prescribed course. At the end of her formulaic collation, Vanessa (who has never met Iris and Cyril), informs Dr T (who has known them both well, for thirty years), that respite care can only be considered after she has been assessed and reported on by 'appropriate' specialist clinics: specifically and separately for her falls, her dementia, her mood instability and her age-related medical complaints. No, there cannot be exceptions. Dr T – almost incredulous, certainly incensed – asks to speak to Vanessa's manager.

There is a delay. When the manager, Marjorie, calls Dr T she seems to be listening diplomatically, but then, equally diplomatically, seems not to have heard or understood. Yes, No. She understands (?) but must support Vanessa in her correct responses: that is how these situations must be managed. Yes, she can understand Dr T's frustration: 'I'm sorry'.

Dr T does not accept defeat. He makes further phone calls. He will shake some senior sense from Social Services, but is told that the regional Director of Social Services is away for two days. He then phones Cyril, whose voice sounds weaker and more short of breath. Dr T asks him about this: Cyril is resigned, self-abnegating, (again) disarmingly accommodating. Dr T refers to administrative delays with respite care: he does not elaborate, but apologises and makes clear he is active in trying to make things happen. 'Yes … Thank you for everything you're doing, doctor … I'll manage somehow.'

But Doctor T does not feel good about this. It is Friday afternoon.

*

On Monday morning Dr T hears. The carer had gone in the previous day and had found both old people on the floor. Iris was moaning with hunger, confusion and soaked underwear, unable to raise herself. Cyril was beside her, but still and silent: grey-mottled and dead. He had probably been trying to lift her.

Iris was immediately taken into care by Social Services.

Dr T feels immersed in an ocean of sadness: for our human frailty, fallibility, folly, pride and evanescence. His surgery is due to start; he dries his eyes.

The whole is more than the sum of its parts.

*

Plans get you into things. But you got to work your way out.

Will Rogers, *The Autobiography of Will Rogers* (1949)

Ω

From Family to Factory

The dying ethos
of personal healthcare

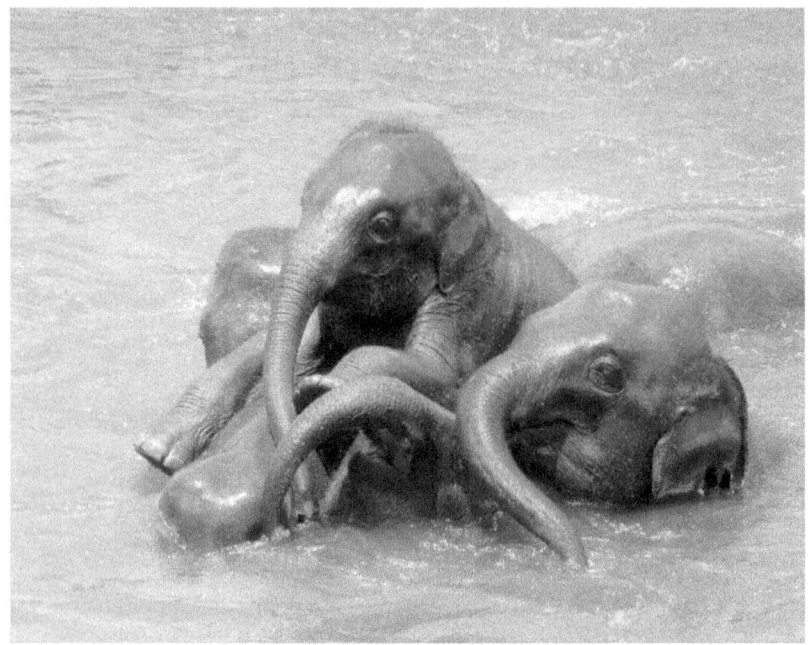

For more than 40 years I have worked as a frontline NHS doctor, mostly as a psychiatrist and GP. With other newswatchers, I join the surges of angry moral revulsion when hearing of the latest exposure of gross neglect of care, or even darker cruelty.

Yet my outrage, sadly, is not shocked: I have long considered such events almost inevitable. For in our eagerness to exploit the efficiencies of industrialisation we have carelessly sacrificed the caring human heart of healthcare. We see 'treatments', but people become invisible. This is – at least sometimes – the price we pay when we create a culture that excessively objectifies and commodifies the complexly human.

I remember a different ethos. At the start of my work in the NHS – before our hermetic rhetoric of measurement, quantification, computer-coding and managed goals and targets – I thought of my working milieu as a (mostly) good-humoured, well-functioning family. Complex tasks were shared across disciplines with welcoming courtesy and cooperation. Roles and experience were sensibly recognised and respected, but rarely rigidly enforced. Likewise inter-professional boundaries: we usually accurately understood others' competence and responsibility and adjusted our activities and encounters accordingly. There was often considerable overlap of skills and practice: this would now be regarded as 'untidy' and inefficient, but actually was usually to everyone's benefit – we could provide a more seamless service: it was easy to refer patients across to colleagues whose work and language we understood, and who were often personally known to us. Although one practitioner might be best suited to a particular task, others could expediently temporise and substitute themselves when necessary: like well-functioning families, where good-faith prevails, this would be guided by open dialogue – by sense and sensibility. The result? Patients rarely got lost within or between systems: personal attachment and knowledge guided a sense of continual care. Practitioners, too, enjoyed this broad conviviality. We can see these principles operating in well-functioning families: the healthy resilience both of the entire group, and its individual members, depends on an ever-changing mixture of structure and flexibility.

In human families there are essential jobs to be done: the 'infrastructure' for the security and welfare of all. But beyond that families exist to play, provide nourishment, pleasure and meaning for one another – and then create new life that transcends and may surprise them all. These life-affirmations all had their equivalents in my first two decades of NHS work. I felt part of a large 'organic' network of care – colleagues then seemed like relatives of many kinds, who also ranged in familiarity, seniority, wisdom and power. There were other subtle fruits from this family-like network of care: we knew and understood real families far better than we do now. I remember many helpful conversations with 'family doctors', helping us understand the struggles, yearnings and sorrows of the ailing within their patients' families. Within this family-sensitive, vast, sprawling NHS 'family' I had myriad and mostly good contacts with my healthcare 'siblings'. I appreciated then – more now – that I was part of one of the best, and most workable, kinds of 'Confederate Socialism'.

*

It was not to last. For the last two decades we have seen a progressive dismantling of this family ethos. Successive think-tanks, management consultants, specialist committees and then briefed-politicians have adopted the mindset of the engineer, the industrialist and the market-economist. Healthcare is now forged as a kind of Civic Engineering or, even, a project for Venture Capitalists. Some forms of healthcare submit well to these approaches: the elimination of Poliomyelitis and the spur to advanced pharmaceuticals are respective examples of clear successes. The treatment of certain well-defined physical illnesses – for example, a the surgical remedy of the blocked coronary artery or opaque eye lens – are now routine 'products' of these approaches.

But we must beware of losing our balance: for our new managed healthcare culture is now evolving more like an insect colony than a human family: roles set rigid, repetitive, prescribed, and dictated. Skills become narrow and executed without either consciousness or view of the whole. Care is reduced to a complex system of interlocking, algorithmically proceduralised tasks: an Airfix Kit of (non) human engagement.

In contrast, a healthy human family is like a garden: growth is facilitated, protected, tended – never coerced. Relationships are nourished and encouraged as ends in themselves, not for any external 'product' (though often this may be spawned). How different this is to our insect-colony-like healthcare factories where all human conduct is mandated and managed by the group's circuit-board. Relationships and communications are subsumed to a strict division of labour – rarely are they ends in themselves. Individual variation is likely to be perceived as subversion. The group's totalitarian function commands all.

Clearly the ethos and activities of the family and the factory both have essential – yet very different – places in our complex lives. This extends to our healthcare. An important task needs to be discerned: the necessity for wise and flexible judgment as to how to balance these opposing principles in all our important human projects. Failures are common. For example, attempting to 'manage' family life by uncompromising parental authority will not work for long: eventually myriad forms of unhappiness, subversion and defiance will obliquely countermand.

Yet, as we have seen, our factory-industrial approach has procured us massive benefits, otherwise unreachable. But, when overused, this approach can alienate, erode and destroy important human bonds and understandings. In healthcare we must be vigilant, for these conundra and complexities demand our endless capacity for fresh and creative compromises.

*

Our factory-type healthcare will deal poorly with those many human ailments that need different kinds of personal engagement for their relief and transcendence. These require healing encounters that mobilise the sufferer's internal resources for immunity, growth and repair. These are subtle and delicate activities and – importantly – cannot develop in a factory culture, whose structure and function both depend on rigidity (like a vehicle chassis). They can only emerge and thrive in a family-type milieu where structure and function and strength are linked to flexibility and elasticity (like a tyre). The general principle for healthcare is that while factory-type management may be best for conduction of less psychologically demanding tasks ('Science'), it is much less suited to socially and psychologically complex situations, where subtle, imaginative induction is required ('Art').

We need these kinds of inductions for any successful attempt to understand personal experience and meaning. For these there are no adequate plans or maps – for while personal experience and distress may contain universal themes, they are always – in some ways – unique. The factory cannot recognise such important discriminations and thus can only hinder us. Yes, our ideas of faulty biomechanics are essential in many of our healthcare encounters but we will often need, also, other approaches of flexibility and imagination. We need some understanding of this person's life, experience , struggles and relationships: holism and semiotics – this is that as well as this. In a culture that is less industrially rigid and driven, the power and meaning of personal attachments will extend far beyond procedures. This is what happens in 'good' families.

*

The price of short-circuiting all this is high: it is what we have now. I am told there is much academic, systematic research into such matters. In my realm – a veteran frontline doctor – what do I experience? I now inhabit a world much richer in precise, high-technology interventions and informatics, and much safer from evident rogue or incompetent practitioners. Yet it is a world more humanly impoverished: of human connection, knowledge, understanding, affection or enduring personal concern. I now attend many meetings with harassed, dead-eyed, fatigued, dispirited doctors. They say: 'I do what I have to', and talk of earliest-date retirement – despite being better remunerated than ever before. Our meetings are pressure-cookers of abstracted management: Agendae, Goals and Targets, budgets, performance indicators, Care Pathways Exception Reporting, Integrated Care – a new lexicon of depersonalised management. It is many years since I sat together with colleagues to better personally understand and develop our frequent and inevitably flawed, fragile and evanescent human work. The factory has driven out the family: I am frustrated and sorrowful. I still have some cohorts: displaced older members of a now-homeless vocational family. We commiserate.

*

What of patients ('service users'!): what do I hear? Those most satisfied – I fear transiently – are those plucked with timely and efficient specialist intervention from cardiovascular or malignant catastrophe: the life-saving coronary artery stent or hemicolectomy. Well-managed factory-healthcare does well here: these beneficial matchings must be acknowledged and continued.

But I hear many more stories of another kind: of vulnerable, fearful people (all of us, sometimes?) feeling personally insignificant, unknown and unanchored in a large, complex, indecipherable system. There is a new kind of anomie in our healthcare: I hear it routinely from intelligent, conscientious, alert people – that they do not know the name of their GP ('The Surgery is so big and busy: I see somebody different each time.'). Likewise the elderly or mentally anguished ('No, I can't remember the name of the clinic or the doctor: there are so many … They said they'll send me another appointment. Yes, I'll do what I'm told …'). From older patients I hear laments for the loss of smaller, friendlier practices and the hospital general physician who saw them through many travails ('Dr X and his staff knew me and my family: I didn't have to explain … I felt understood and cared for …'). Wanting to continue my ethos of family doctor, I frequently extend my interest and the interview, to develop better personal understanding. Younger patients are surprised – positively and appreciatively ('No one before has shown the interest to speak with me like this.'). As a family doctor this was easy: it is much more difficult as a 'primary-care service provider'.

*

The ennui and fractious demoralisation of our NHS has become a constant back-drone in our national life. Periodically we can expect interruptions: startled shrieks from many more sickening healthcare atrocities. These will usually occur within forests of managing regulations and procedures. In the shocked tumult, listen for the displacing, buttressing countercharge: 'Inadequate resources!'.

I do not usually believe this. The impoverishment is of another kind.

*

Healthcare is a humanity guided by science.

Ω

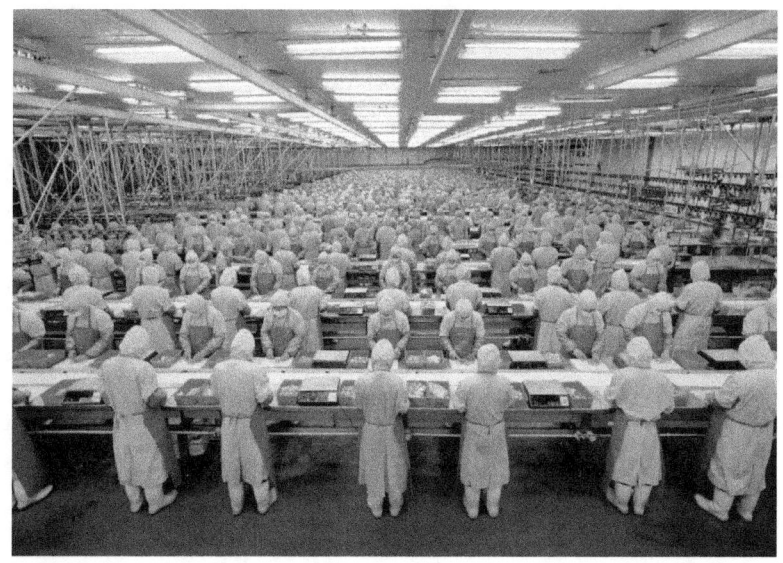

Understanding the Other
Four Elemental Questions for
Therapeutic Psychology

A personal view

Psychology in healthcare faces a conundrum. By entering an arena dominated by the Medical Model it adopts particular types of language, theories and schemata. This it does to be able to 'trade' within the dominant medical 'currency'. Yet such attempts to designate and objectify often displace views and contacts that are more personal, naturalistic, holistic and effective. Thus, the overly academic and technical will frequently miss *this* person and situation. The following, written by a veteran frontline NHS doctor, offers a brief introductory analysis and restitution.

For more than forty years I have had long and short-term responsibilities for myriad forms of human distress presenting to the NHS: as a psychiatrist, psychotherapist and General Practitioner. Throughout this time there has been no shortage of schemata – analytical or interventive – to explain, designate, guide, sometimes enforce. These have changed with the era and the healthcare sector. At times I have wished to pursue and explore these; at other times I have been instructed or commanded, a reluctant recipient. All the mental health schemata have had partial and conditional truth: such fragile connections with human complexity may offer help in attunement, but folly (or worse) when ill-judged. How, then, do we decide? Again, there is no shortage of experts offering more schemes, to direct our decisions. Superficially, this may seem reassuring. Yet I do not think our best judgements readily emerge from such 'authoritative' attempts to objectify and systematise. Our creative discretion is often better served by other perspectives: those that are both more holistic and – simultaneously and subtly – more flexibly personal, more imaginatively bespoke.

What are these perspectives, and how to they escape subsumption to pre-packaged, designatory psychologies? What else can guide our understanding of others and their distress? In my working lifetime I have found the following four questions[1] primal to any likely successful engagement:

- What is it like to be this other person, to have lived their life?
- What is the meaning and experience, for them, of this story and this distress?
- What is the meaning and experience, for them, of me, now?
- What do I need to understand of their needs that they possibly cannot yet express, or even think about?

---

[1] Zigmond, D (2012), 'Five Executive Follies: How commodification imperils compassion in personal healthcare.' *Journal of Holistic Healthcare* Vol 8, Issue 3, December

These questions lie behind and beyond all systematic therapeutic psychologies. They are more fundamental: if a scheme or intervention cannot answer these questions, my engagement is unlikely to be therapeutic, though – paradoxically – it may bring me consonance and belonging among my colleagues. Conversely, sometimes schematic and systematic psychologies can help answer the four questions, though not schematically!

The four questions are 'naïve': unlike our schematic or designatory psychologies, they assume little. Because of this they are more likely to lead to personal understanding that has vernacular qualities, rather than the generic and abstracted nature of more conventional, objectifying psychologies:

'T has never recovered from the childhood terror and sorrow of his experience of father's raging cruelty, brutality, then final desertion. T's life has been spent yearning for, but mistrusting, male support, esteem, affection and affiliation. My lateness for his appointment seems to stir in him intolerable ancient residues of vulnerability, uncertainty and abandonment. His response to my greeting is staccato, flushed and tense: he seems angry and afraid. I sense a conflation of fight and flight and I think, again, of his wounded early childhood.'

Contrast this with:

'T has a long history of recurrent agitated depressive illnesses with anxiety/panic reactions. He had a poor record of maintaining work and long-term relationships. He also has problems with anger management: this was evident to the Clinic Staff when I was unavoidably delayed. This inconvenience was clearly explained to T, who nevertheless was unacceptably angry and rude to the staff in response. It is thus likely that T also has a Personality Disorder.'

The first account is guided by the Four Elemental Questions, the latter by currently conventional designatory notions. Both have their strengths and uses. Optimal practice often comes from a skilful blend. Throughout my decades of practice, though, I have usually found the former to be the more illuminating and helpful. Disturbingly, the necessary engendering ethos – of evocative personal understanding – is now increasingly imperilled: our excessive attempts to standardise and industrialise NHS healthcare have led to a culture where the designatory will thrive and the resonant will perish.

More than a century ago, well before we had become so lost in our forests of systemised abstractions, here is Mark Twain: 'One learns peoples through the heart, not the eyes or the intellect.'[2] Evidently this is only partially true and from another age, but there is pithy wisdom here that is probably more urgently relevant to our times than his. The message in this ancient and folksy voice could help us reclaim our collective sense.

Mental healthcare is a humanity (sometimes) guided by science.

Ω

---

[2] Twain, Mark (1895), 'What Paul Bourget Thinks of Us.' *North American Review*, January

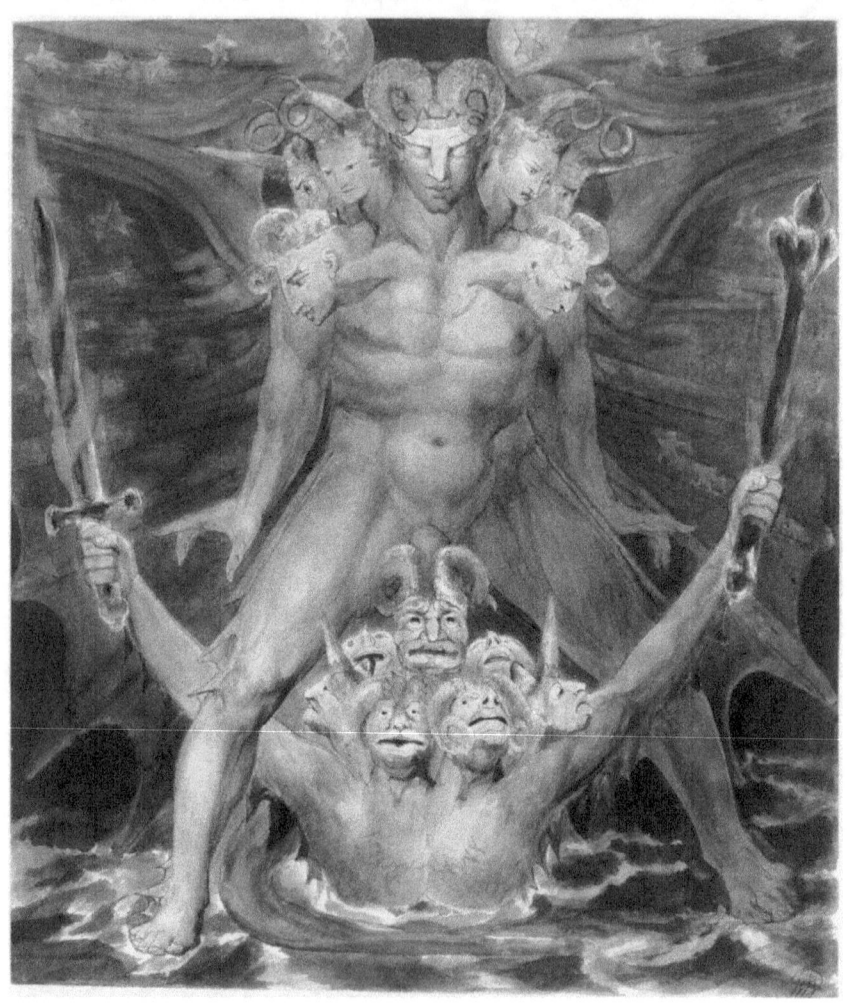

William Blake *The Great Red Dragon and the the Beast from the Sea* 1805-10

Words and Numbers Servants or Masters?

Caveats for holistic healthcare
Part I

Holism's fuller engagement with realities is an aspiration and ideal. It can never be complete, and in practice, there are many obstructions. These range from our use of language to our highly managed and industrialised culture. How does this happen? What are the consequences? This is the first of two articles.

Prologue: caveats for holistic healthcare

Holism (and its lack) may be easier to recognise than define. It is more readily communicated and perceived by stories, rather than data or abstract formulations. This presents problems: holistic mindsets are now becoming harder to access and maintain, for our culture is now one that increasingly conceives and conveys in packages: food, fuel, news, entertainment, even thought are all likely to be coded, metered, monitored, measured or packed. This causes fewer problems when our encounters are with inanimate or less complex life-forms: the production and distribution of eggs or detergents cause fewer ethical and social conundrae than the industrialisation of complex welfare activities (though even our simpler activities eventually confront us with wider ecological – ultimately Gaian – consequences).

We thus have an insoluble handicap. It is always easier to think in parts than wholes: language, analytical thinking, our micro and macro economies … all tend to fragment our perceptions and activities: 'this is this, and that is that'. In contrast, holism's tenet of infinite and often hidden interconnectedness tends to erase boundaries and conflate territories: 'this is that as well as this'. Such thinking largely eludes schemes, packaging, academia, economic analyses. Our use of language, too, struggles to convey any sense of holism without serious loss or distortion.

The following two articles present a collage of notions illustrating, very partially, the extent of our difficulties and task. The notions themselves are presented without usual conventions of academic thoroughness or cohesion. The first article presents the skeleton of the view: the second provides further illustrations and variations. Overall, they represent some unsystematised, though summative, personal reflections from one practitioner's decades of working in human healthcare – a chimeric and often paradoxical world. Philosophical contention is ever-present. We are accelerating our mandates for factory-like language and procedures to service increasingly complex healthcare: human nature and predicaments remain considerably more ambiguous.

1. I've got a measurement – it must be a fact

The rise of data and the curse of scientism

'Nothing vast enters the lives of mortals without a curse'

Sophocles (c 496-405 BC)

There was life and technical success before computers, yet these are rapidly becoming harder to understand. Some examples: the manufacture of antibiotics, the D-Day Landings, Man on the Moon, Concorde – all of these were achieved with minuscule or no computer-power – things we could not manage now in our 'progress'. We have become empowered but deskilled: in healthcare, as we shall see, these subtle discrepancies lead to grievous losses.

Before the widespread use of computers, the harvesting and collation of measurements – data – was manual, labour-intensive and therefore slow. It thus required much deliberation and discrimination and – relative to today – its volume was tiny and consequently much more manageable.

The electronic unshackling of these activities has freed them from the constraints of our individual capacities for engagement, assimilation or understanding: data has multiplied exponentially and is now pumped and piped at us like gas or water – public commodities.

Measurement, the blood-brother of data, has thus been conferred pre-eminent status in many humanly-complex activities. Numbers are the most easily digested 'food' for computers, and computers are now essential to the functioning of any public service. Existence of people and their activities must be continually monitored and broadcast in a form that can ensure their organisational recognition, management and survival. The virtual world now defines and commands the real: measure or perish. Once started, this is difficult to slow or stop.

So, our institutions are now electronically held together by computers, computers need data, data need statistics, statistics need measurements; ergo: measurement becomes the basic language and activity.

What does this mandatory measurement mean for healthcare? The consequences vary greatly with the type of activity. Sometimes the effect is facilitating and benign. For example, with activities that can be easily and directly measured, standardised and proceduralised: here the measurement culture can be applied with relative ease and evident benefit. Laboratory services, vaccinations and cataract extractions all serve as common examples. All have in common a clear, circumscribed physical basis, little variation in technique or human response and a high completion/success rate. In short, they can be easily humanly 'mechanised'.

But much of healthcare does not offer this kind of simplicity for measurement, and then the effects often depart widely from the benign and facilitative. Measurements are at their most competent with physical objects or phenomena: a blood-count is far less problematic or contentious than a mood-rating scale. This is because attempts to assess, measure and code other people's experiences must be derived from something else: self-reports, or other people's perception being the commonest. All are subject to massive contention, contamination and compromise. What does this mean? Here are some personalised examples:

Ms B is in dispute with the Department for Work and Pensions (DWP)[1] over her Disability Living Allowance. Ms B claims severe symptoms and invalidity from Depression, but her invalidity seems invalid to the DWP assessor: he asks the GP, Dr F, for his opinion. Dr F[2], in a complex but rapid judgement, agrees with the assessor. This 'objective' assessment is stymied by Ms B's continually high self-reported, but quantified, depression scores. 'Something's wrong' they all say in different ways. 'Only the wearer knows where the shoe pinches' says an old adage, but when is this untrue? Who decides? How?

Kenny is sixty-two years old, a single, lonely man, appeasing and self-deprecating in his manner. Harsh and neglectful parenting left him with impoverished self-esteem. A working lifetime as a road worker has riddled his lower body with degenerative arthritis. He left school at fourteen: his intelligence exceeds his words. After several years of courteous wariness he is, with Dr F's gentle encouragement, beginning to talk of his burden of fear, loneliness, shame and longing. The ancient story behind it is poignant and powerful. Kenny has great faith in Dr F, but continues anguished in his small and crumbling world. Dr F asks for help from NHS Psychological Services, to help Kenny occupy his limited life more positively. Kenny returns to Dr F a fortnight later, fearful, tearful and trembling. He nervously indicates the immediate cause of his distress: a tightly-stuffed, freshly opened envelope. It is from the Psychology Services. Dr F surveys several detailed questionnaires[3] aiming to define diagnosis, severity, disability and numerous personal and demographic details. In addition are various bureaucratically prolix letters and documents explaining 'The Service', a Complaints Procedure and instructions for the Service User. No one has spoken to him

In his frightened and faltering language Kenny conveys to Dr F his sense of bewildered humiliation and abject inadequacy: 'I don't understand all this, doctor … I just can't do it … I just want to talk to someone – like I do with you, doctor.

The doctor remembers many years ago reading of Heisenberg, an early 20th century physicist. Heisenberg found that it was impossible to plot simultaneously the velocity and locus of an electron without changing these in an indeterminate way: the observation changed the reality. Dr F as a young man could not identify how this was relevant to his meagre knowledge of physics. Many years later he is seeing clearly how personal observation – when formulaic and non-bespoke – can adversely affect people he knows well.

Philip is eighty-six and Dr F is visiting him at home, the week after his discharge from hospital. He had taken a first-ever overdose of his medication to end his life. An earlier than expected visit from his carer had found him collapsed and vomiting.

Philip now looks tired and Dr F again senses immense melancholia beneath the mask of rigid discipline, of understatement. The doctor knows some of Philip's recent trials and sorrows: his wife's gruelling and fatal malignant illness, followed rapidly by the sudden death of his beloved son, their only child. And then the increasing impoverishment of his own Parkinson's Disease, a gathering bass-note.

Dr F had premonitioned Philip's trapped but mute anguish and its possible tragic fruition, and had asked for help from his mental health services. Their (non) engagement proceeded by asking Philip to fill in detailed mood and anxiety questionnaires. These indicated mild, stable disturbance – measurements meriting merely a brief psychological care package from a Low Intensity (skills?) Worker, and a routine, templated report of all this, electronically conveyed to Dr F.

Dr F's perception is discrepant. He shares his unease with Philip, whose intelligence and insight survive his ravages of grief: 'I don't like to tell anyone my troubles, doctor ... I wasn't brought up like that. I have my pride, you know ... It's different with you: I've known you years, and I don't have to say much, for you to understand. But answer all those questions for a stranger? No.'

Dr F thinks of Philip's formative years: a harsher, crueller, braver world of much greater trials, losses and endurance; a black-and-white world where contained and stoic fortitude was a social essential. Dr F understands this with few words, and Philip understands that he understands. But a questionnaire?

Yet Dr F now inhabits a professional world in thrall to designated experts who are keen to quickly code and quantify the distress of Philip and Kenny, as well as Dr F's ministrations, and then to instruct them all. Dr F's understanding can seem piecemeal, slow and never finished: features of the intersubjective, one-person-and-situation-at-a-time. By contrast the questionnaire has slick allure: its 'objectivity' may be specious, but it is quantifiable and can be given to all – a demotic science. Dr F is thinking of the distinction between the scientific and the scientistic: which is which? He is thinking, too, beyond his own professional end: who then will be speaking to the Philips of the world, and what kind of conversations will they be?

*

2. I've got a word – it must be real

The trap of reification

'In the Beginning was the Word'

John 1:1 (date uncertain)

Language does far more than merely 'communicate': words first contain, then command and control our experience, and then our influence of others. The implications of this for healthcare are subtle, powerful and rarely discussed. A brief linguistic analysis will help us understand these.

All words are there to package and convey a description of, or notion about, human experience. All ultimately come from our perceptions, then our constructions. The basic components of language are: adjectives, describing qualities of experience (what something is like); verbs, describing activity producing change (what something does); and nouns, which attempt to capture a more static state, a 'something', from which these other two emanate (what something 'is'). For example, I describe a small vertical platform supported by four vertical supporting posts: someone comes and sits on it – it is a 'chair'. Generally, we think such 'real' things endure and we attribute them by nouns: adjectives and verbs are more the flux of experience

In our usual waking life this may present few problems, with nouns seamlessly providing apposite bridges and anchors for the rest of our sense-experience, and those of others. But potential dislocation is ever-present.

An example: I am at a friend's table, eating an unfamiliar dish. I do not recognise the texture or flavour of the meat, although I enjoy both. I enquire what 'it' is.

1. I am told: 'It is lamb'. I am mellow with appreciation for my sensations, my friend and the cosmos.

2. I am told: 'It is Alginon, my ginger cat. She was very old and was dying anyway'. What is in my mouth now triggers an explosion of nausea, and retching. I jump up with disgust and mistrust. My friend and the cosmos turned malign.

The 'actual' experience is transformed by the idea of the 'real' source-object (lamb v cat). This noun now determines my subsequent experience and action: the adjectives (pleasure or revulsion) and the verbs (sitting and eating v jumping up and retching). All this happens despite my never seeing the putative lamb or cat: they are abstractions rendered powerfully 'real' by the noun. Such is the power and gravitational force of nouns.

Nouns work with greatest clarity and efficiency when applied to physical objects: the words 'table' or 'television' rarely cause problems except to a foreigner, a lawyer or certain kinds of academic. We generally accept these object-nouns as 'real'. Elsewhere the use of nouns is more problematic and more interesting: God, democracy or love may sound like (sacred) 'things', yet are essentially variegated ideas. Innumerable stories from world or domestic histories show how little clarity and consensus the nouns manage here, yet how real they are to their believers.

There are striking analogies in healthcare. One working definition of medical diagnosis is the organisation, then transformation of adjectives (a) and verbs (v) into professionally conferred nouns (n) which then determine explanation, therapeutic action and prediction for others. With afflictions that are predominantly physical – 'structural pathology' or disease – we can call this type of noun a 'Substantial Diagnosis'. Here is a simple example:

Tommy is six. Last night he became listless (a), pushed away (v) his favourite supper, complained of soreness (a) in his throat and abdomen and then started to shiver and vomit (v). Dr Y is now with Tommy and his mother. His job is to find and then confer the right organising noun, or diagnosis. When he sees Tommy's much enlarged, reddened tonsils, flecked with creamy pus, he has the precise constellated noun: 'Acute Pustular Tonsillitis', though he thinks 'Tonsillitis' sufficient for his verbal communications. The formulation and conveyance of this word are beneficial for all: Dr Y knows what to do and what to expect, Tommy will almost certainly get better, Mother is comforted by this and the containing, reassuring clarity of this noun – the Substantial Diagnosis. For all, this process is helpful and uncontentious: the doctor's knowing and naming the 'thing' of Tonsillitis is a cooperative and shared blessing. Importantly, Dr

Y's diagnosis also relieves the sufferers from having to search for their own explanation, meaning of, or influence on, events.

In other areas of healthcare this hegemonic use of nouns runs into many more difficulties. This is particularly so where the doctor is dealing with bodily dysfunction (functional disease) in the absence of the evident structural changes of bodily disease. Equal difficulties are encountered with disorders of behaviour, appetite, mood or impulse (BAMI): the core of psychiatry and clinical psychology. The results here are more mixed: our medical-noun type diagnosis may sometimes bring evident clarity and relief to these physically non-fixated forms of distress, but often it will not. Then the professionally conferred noun – the diagnosis – is conveyed, but the benefits do not follow. In these situations the diagnosis may be 'correct', but clarification, relief or prediction remain poor. The doctor has – by convention – done his job, but none of the participants are gratified. We can call this a 'Nominal Diagnosis'. Here are two examples:

K, a tense, conscientious, sensitive woman of twenty-six years has seen several doctors over several years with benign abdominal and bowel symptoms. All have agreed she has Irritable Bowel Syndrome (IBS) and prescribed the usual medications, always with little or transient effect. Dr T realises that a wider vocabulary is needed to differently understand and influence her complaints. In his endeavour to do this, he learns a lot about her unhappy childhood home and how this has led to her guarded perfectionism and her painful ambivalence about close relationships. The long-term effects of this widened dialogue and vocabulary were slowly gratifying for both K and her doctor.

Here the conventional noun-diagnosis of IBS was relatively ineffective and – probably – obscuring or obstructing more helpful personal understanding: it thus proved to be a Nominal

Diagnosis only. The idiomorphic understanding she developed with Dr T proved much more helpful.

Maggie, fifty-five years, has collected a variety of diagnoses from her many years of faltering contact with psychiatrists and psychologists: Generalised Anxiety Disorder, Agoraphobia, Panics, Emotionally Unstable Personality Disorder with Cyclothymia, Recurrent Depressive Disorder, Bipolar Affective Disorder. All are documented in the usual formalised language of designatory healthcare which then rhetorically confine and define Maggie by Nominal Diagnoses. These conferred nouns may superficially appear to offer real therapeutic understanding, leverage and prediction, but actually do not. None have offered Dr V. greater personal understanding of Maggie.

Dr V. decides to create a larger and different kind of space for Maggie to talk. This dramatically changes not only Dr V.'s view and understanding of Maggie, but also Maggie's behaviour: her symptoms become much quietened.

How does this happen? Dr V. wants to know Maggie's story, not for a Management Plan, but so that he can better understand. Her story has obscurely disturbed her for decades and it will disturb Dr V. now.

Twenty-five years ago she was married – happily she thought – with three children. She experienced her husband as kind, attractive and funny, but a bit feckless: he drank a lot. She suddenly has unmistakable evidence of his alcoholically hazed, repeated sexual contact with their ten-year-old daughter, Amanda. In a volcanic eruption of mixed and primitive feelings, her marriage and family are destroyed. Years later the ruined landscape of her life is still littered with explosives. She tells Dr V. of a current torment: Amanda – now a tough, cynical, sexually alluring, drug-abusing, spiky thirty-four year old single mother – has restored affectionate contact with her father and his second wife, and takes her children to see them.

Maggie's feelings towards her daughter are raw, kaleidoscopic and irresolvable: 'My mind goes crazy with it, doctor ... She was only ten: I should have known, should have protected her: but she knew, and she knew that I didn't know ... She was a child, but was – I didn't know then – a serious sexual rival. Now she is stronger and healthier than me, and has more of a family – mine is destroyed. I love her as a mother, but hate her for what she did, what she does, what they have all done: but can I blame her? ... Has she triumphed over me? I feel crazy and terrible for having just said all that, doctor, yet it's such a relief that I can say these things and that you can understand ...'

Dr V. has a bespoke and ongoing dialogue with Maggie about her tragic story and her responses to it. Her distress often exceeds her capacity for words, yet words and ideas are what they exchange and they are many: guilt, shame, loss, rage, hate, love, contrition, resentment, despair, despondency, alienation, disconnection, blame, humiliation, revenge, sorrow, defeat ... All touch on part of Maggie's poisoned cauldron, but only part, and only transiently. Maggie now talks less of her symptoms and Dr V. does not much offer his vocabulary of diagnoses or treatments. As their language has changed, so has the nature of their exchange, and then the pattern of Maggie's distress. Maggie, so long burdened and defined by her multi-diagnoses, is now freer to suffer with her unique and humanly-understood tragedy. Dr V., too, though distressed by her story, is also touched and, paradoxically, nourished by such candid and courageous contact – the staple of compassion.

Others have asked: what is 'really' wrong with Maggie? Is there a word: is it 'Depression'? What is the 'correct treatment'?

'Language is, by its very nature a communal thing: that is, it expresses never the exact thing, but a compromise – that which is common to you, me and everybody.'

Thomas Ernest Hulme (1923), *Romanticism and Classical Speculations*

This article continues in chapter 2.17 If you want good personal healthcare see a Vet.

*

Notes

1) DWP – a UK nationwide governmental department that administers and manages state pensions, sickness and welfare benefits etc. Assessing disputed levels of distress and disability is a task it currently often subcontracts to other agencies.

2) The doctors, patients and situations throughout this article are real but anonymised. The examples of doctors' encounters will be relevant now to many other types of healthcare professionals, especially those working for the NHS or large corporations.

3) Detailed questionnaires are now being vaunted and proceduralised throughout most NHS Psychology and Counselling Services. This is explained by authorities as making the services more scientifically efficient. This is contentious, at least. In this author's view it leads to specious science, dehumanisation, and a healthcare cult of Scientism. The obstructive and destructive effect of these is extensive and subtle. See my articles 'How to Help Harry' (Zigmond, 2012) and 'Sense and Sensibility' (Zigmond, 2011a).

References

Zigmond, D (2012) *How to Help Harry – Friend or Foe? The scientific and the scientistic in the fog of the frontline*
Zigmond, D (2011a) *Sense and Sensibility: The danger of Specialisms to holistic, psychological care*

Ω

Publ. in *Journal of Holistic Healthcare Vol 10 Issue 3 2013*

If you want
good personal healthcare,
see a Vet

Caveats for holistic healthcare
Part II

The over-explicit and over-schematic can block our perception of larger and more subtle realities. This second of two articles explores further how this happens, and what we may be left with.

The fairest thing we can experience is the mysterious. It is the fundamental emotion which stands at the cradle of true art and science.

Albert Einstein (1934), *The World as I see It*

1. Never invade Russia!

This was Churchill's droll, jesting yet ominous response to an enquiry about his most crucial guiding military maxim.

Napoleon and Hitler are the best-known examples of Churchill's warnings of epic folly: maelstroms of shocking, humbled hubris. Both launched their expeditions fresh from success in easier campaigns and fuelled by specious optimism. They were driven also by rhetoric for the rightness and feasibility for the possession of new territory. Both started with startling triumphalism, then slowed, then succumbed: exhausted by the vastness and strangeness of a climate, terrain and people they had poorly understood.

There are useful analogies for some of our current enervating endeavours and conundra in healthcare. First, our expectations have been primed and inflated: Life for millions in the Twentieth Century was positively transformed by applied science. Biomedicine has had spectacular success in countering, even eliminating, many infectious, inflammatory and degenerative physical diseases. In all this, industrialisation – mass-production, standardisation, quantification, speed – has been essential. Such successes have led to a long flush of optimism: surely we can gainfully apply similar schematic, industrial-medical type thinking and interventions to *all* our other sources of distress and pain – our human dis-ease, our polymorphous anguish, our inevitable (yes, still!) decline?

It is here that our invincible march founders, for ailments of our metaphorical heart are proving far harder to locate, define or reverse than those of our anatomical heart. Human motivation, meaning, communication and (un)consciousness yield very meagre territories to objectifying science. Beyond is our vast hinterland, navigable (sometimes) by other kinds of knowledge and influence.

Our reluctance to heed this accounts for many of our most curious and (superficially) indecipherable healthcare follies. In our thrall to measurement we neglect more important unmeasurables. In our urge to treat we do not pause to heal. In our (often unnecessary) compulsion to convergently image the part, we become blind to the divergent – the whole: *this* person, their story and networks. When we define, we also often confine – ourselves and others – to a tunnelled vision and selective deafness. For language, perception and action are tightly linked. If the language of our culture becomes restricted to the technical, the commercial, the procedural and the defined, then our patients – people, like us! – are seen as merely biomechanical problems to be controlled, managed, traded or disposed of. The abstract becomes hegemonic: the real become abstract.

Hyperbole?

Even in 'straightforward' physical care our over-industrialisation is producing shocking calumnies. Consider the following story recently widely reported in the media:[1]

A man is admitted to a London Hospital with a rare but well recognised physical complaint (Diabetes Insipidus) which renders him particularly and hazardously vulnerable to dehydration. He knows this and can usually communicate well. He is seen and assessed by a succession of healthcare workers, some of them specialists. In their complexly successive, jigsawedly interlocking, brief contacts with him they do not heed this increasingly desperate requests for water, which culminate in his calling 999 from the hospital ward. Only after he dies does it become clear that all these algorithmically-managed practitioners had been effectively deaf to his voice and blind to his demeanour. Hospital spokespersons' public comments are woven with grave contrition and confusion. The former might need construction, the latter does not. The Hospital used to have world-renown for its standards of medical practice, teaching and academia; emblematised also by its historic, stately architecture. Relocated now in an undistinguished, unloved, ugly, airport-like, sprawling conurbation, the containing architecture expresses with unintended accuracy the healthcare culture – a hive of hired healthdroids.

That a highly-funded, well equipped and specialised *medical* unit can so misunderstand and depersonalise someone with a *physical* complaint can only bode poorly elsewhere – especially for those who require yet more personal and thoughtful kinds of listening and understanding. This is the case, but often less obvious. With non-physical complaints our failures of care and communication are less dramatic: a slow slide into lonely and dislocated oblivion will gather no headlines. Living silently with a broken-heart attracts no crowds; an untimely death from a heart attack does.

Our current healthcare is in increasing thrall to a Scientistic folly: that generic formulations can be mass produced for all individual distress – that human dis-ease can thus be easily subsumed to impersonally managed forms of civic engineering. Such is contemporary healthcare's Invasion of Russia: grandiose but flawed in assumption, then unsustainable, impossible and incurring vast casualties.[2]

Healthcare may be guided by our science, but science must rarely eclipse our humanity.

*

2. If you want good personal healthcare, see a Vet

'I like peasants – they are not sophisticated enough to reason speciously'

Montesquieu (1689-1755), *Variétés*

When Dr F takes his dog to the Vet, Mo, he is simultaneously disarmed, comforted, ashamed and envious: Mo has a guileless and effortless rapport and liking for the animals she is handling. Dr F wants to know more of these unaffected and unbookish skills: he asks to sit in with her.

What Dr F witnesses is humbling and radically refreshing. After asking the owner a few questions, Mo stands back from the animal, scanning it with her eyes, listening carefully to its breathing and other sounds. Then she makes active contact with the animal, the approach being based, Dr F thinks, on some kind of 'holistic mind-set' that she senses the animal is now inhabiting. Dr F notices how different her approaches are: with one she gazes at its face with unwavering directness while speaking in a firm and commanding voice; with the next she averts her gaze, softens her posture and lowers her voice to a soft reticence. Sometimes she quickly and directly grasps the nape of the neck with decisive dominance, a wordless control. At others she is slow and light of touch, gently stroking the flank while humming; a trans-species fraternalism. Dr F wonders whether Mo's accuracy, range and speed of rapport with these different creatures is somehow akin to inducing hypnotic states in humans. He asks Mo:

'Oh, I don't know about hypnosis – I'm not that clever. Nor do I know much about humans: they talk too much for me to be able to understand them!' She curls a playfully commiserating look at Dr F. 'My furry friends here can't say much, but I have to understand them quickly: are they frightened, hungry, confused, in pain, angry, unloved? ... Yes, really! ... Do they need to feel they still control their territory, or do they need to know I am dominant? All such things I have to get right

231

without much delay, otherwise I cannot get docility enough to do my job ... Yes, I'll get scratched and bitten, too. With larger animals it can be more serious: you can easily become lunch or squash!'.

Dr F leaves Mo that morning with a deeper gratitude than he is easily able to express. With little psychological scholarship, theory or instruction, this open-hearted, open-minded, freshly-instinctive woman is able to resonate with, and thus 'read', the mind-set of these (humanly) mute creatures. What natural gifts we (all?) may have!

He thinks of the cumbersome, academically conceived, elaborate-yet-clumsy devices healthcare workers are being instructed to use, to inform all about the experience – the 'mental state' – of others. He thinks of the obedient but hopeless Scientism of giving detailed questionnaires to Kenny and Philip[3]. He then thinks of Mo: her almost wordless, seemingly magical, rapid and affectionate rapport with very different animals. He wishes he could be understood like that, and laughs to himself. His laughter diffuses to a smile at the contrasted memories: Mo has inspired him to retrieve some fresh depth and contact in his work. He will reconnect with himself too, before and beyond words.

*

3. In difficult encounters, think about sex

The tyranny of the explicit

'Every person's feelings have a front-door and a side-door by which they may be entered.'

Oliver Wendell Holmes Sr, *The Autocrat of the Breakfast Table* (1858)

Dr Y is thinking about sex. It is not the first time, but now it is different. He is thinking professional thoughts about how our thinking and behaviour around our sexuality could greatly enlighten our healthcare.

More specifically, Dr Y is thinking about a very delicate, complex and evanescent interweaving – of the implicit and the explicit: how these have to be rapidly and accurately discerned, deciphered, jointly understood and then responded to. All of this happens on a second by second basis. And choreographing this medley of meta-communications is essential for any kind of sexual competence – let alone deeper unifying satisfactions. We have to have a (usually) unspoken sense of what the other is desirous of, receptive to, 'on' for, and when and how. We must quickly sense error and redirection. Mostly, in better sexual congress, this can happen by dextrous implicit exchanges: the explicit may sometimes then be added potently and sparingly – a mutual aphrodisiac. If the explicit is necessary, the exchange is faltering. If it is necessary for long periods, the relationship is in serious trouble. If the explicit is used by one, without implicit desire by the other, the exchange becomes embarrassed, self-consciously clumsy, possibly abortive. Many such misattunements doom a relationship. Seriously regarded, they can become work for lawyers.

Dr Y is amusing and confusing himself with how weighty and complicated are the responsibilities of this ancient[4] and near universal activity. How do most of us ever (think we) get it right?

These implicit-explicit dances are certainly at the heart of our sexual contacts, but extend throughout our important relationships. They depend on our being able to seamlessly interchange the implicit and explicit, by 'tuning-in' to the other. We want (and expect) our partner to understand what is troubling us, without our having to name it (yet?): soon after, we want them to now be receptive to the beginnings (or resumption) of the explicit. We want, now, to be able to talk. Yes, directly.

Familiar?

Dr Y extends his thinking to how important such exchanges are in healthcare. He remembers Maggie's[3] long story and considers how any success he has with her is due to his being mindful of such delicate dances: he had been patiently implicit with her before she trusted him with the explicit. And then, with gratified relief, her healing reverted to the implicit. Maggie had told Dr Y of earlier psychiatric interviews and how they had become too explicit too rapidly. She had retreated to the shelter of the implicit, but had not been understood. The implicit locked.

Dr Y remembers well the kinds of discussions he used to have with colleagues, at the beginning of his career. He recalls many years of interrupted-but-never-finished, free-wheeling explorations of our complex contact with others. The concepts and vocabulary were rich and wide: influence, confluence, identity, boundaries, encryption, territory, projection, surrender, escape ... The notions and vocabulary were plastic and uncompletable, yet each alightment could enrich – differently in different conversations: subtly or evidently, with immediacy or incubation, with implicity or explicity.

Dr Y now rarely has such polychromatic and rewarding exchanges. The computer has predicated a new healthcare language for the 21st century: a restricted and restrictive machine-mandated vocabulary. Healthcarers communicate now – almost entirely – in dull narrow administrative, technical words: of conventions, clusters and codes; of quantifiable procedural activity and description; of conduction but not induction – all designating the objectively generic but excluding the humanly variable. Computer compatibility may thus build some bridges to our outer lives, but very few to our inner. What remains has little room for the nascent, the semiotic, the metamorphic, the ambiguous – all the subtle hues that we must mindfully respect to provide nourishment and meaning for our important relationships. The explicit now burgeons beyond our needs, understanding, tolerance or stamina: the implicit ails and dies.

*

Its passing takes much of us, too.

*

The whole is more than the sum of its (explicit) parts.

*

Healthcare is a humanity guided by science.

*

Humanity may be commanded by the explicit: its best understanding is often implicit.

*

'The water in the vessel is sparkling; the water in the sea is dark. The small truth has words that are clear; the great truth has great silence.'

Rabindranath Tagore, *Stray Birds* (1916)

Notes

[1] It is hard to gain statistics about the human and economic cost of inflexible, officious practice and uncompassionate – if 'correct' – depersonalised care. What correlates does one measure? Who is going to fund this? Although quantitative research may be difficult to set up, vernacular evidence is plentiful and ubiquitous. See my articles 'Five Executive Follies' (Zigmond, 2011b) and 'Love's Labour's Lost' (Zigmond, 2010). Also letters to Clinical Directors of Mental Health Services.

[2] Kane Gorny, age twenty-two, died on 25 May 2009 of dehydration as an in-patient at St George's Hospital, south London. The inquest in July 2012 revealed the facts recorded here. The story is only one of several similar in recent years, eg see also reports of Mid Staffs and West Midlands NHS Trusts. All have been met with convulsions of outraged incomprehension when made public. The fact that they come clearly to public view reflects well on investigative journalism but – of course – seriously damages confidence in NHS care. This is rendered more confusing when such episodes occur in institutions deemed to be 'performing' excellently by other, measured criteria. The responses of managerial gravitas, concern and contrition seem real enough. Some sceptics have averred that these conceal some kind of collusion, albeit unconscious. The latter possibility is easier to cite and sense than see. If true, this is cultural: powerful, but difficult to tether or examine, except by inference.

[3] Kenny, Philip and Maggie are all real but anonymised victims of over-schematised and over-explicit mental healthcare. Their encounters with Dr Y are described in the previous article 'Words and Numbers: Servants or Masters?'

[4] The activity itself is much older than many people realise. For example, this author – together with many of his generation – believed they were its initiators in the 1960s. However, since that time there has been increasing evidence from many sources, indicating that it far predates that period – possibly even prior to the birth of this author's own parents.

References

Zigmond, D. (2011b) *Five Executive Follies: How commodification imperils compassion in personal healthcare*
Zigmond, D. (2010) *Psychiatry Love's Labour Lost: The pursuit of The Plan and the eclipse of the personal*

Publ. in *Journal of Holistic Healthcare* Vol II Issue 1 2014

Democratic Fatigue - Information Overload

So, few people seem interested in electing a Police Commissioner. Soon after, the media parade for us politicians, academics and pundits – all expressing perplexity or concern. One recurring salvaging explanation is that citizens do not have enough information to make a choice.

As one of these unengaged citizens, I do not share these puzzlements, concerns or notions. My mind and life are overwhelmed by choices and information, and I cannot cope with more. There is a great difference between wanting to have an individual voice and access to dialogue, and submitting to governmentally initiated and designed choice of other people's packages. I may want the many authorities in my life to listen, but I do not want, necessarily, the responsibility of having to vet or choose who all those authorities might be. Evolved democracy is very different from democracy by government prescription.

There are interesting parallels here to our current healthcare commissioning. As a senior GP I know most of my peers have little enthusiasm for their freshly bestowed mantle of authority: Clinical Commissioning Groups. Yes, we want managers to listen, but we do not want to have to do their job. Putatively democratised devices to commission Welfare Services appeal to certain kinds of politicians, academics and tank-thinkers. But those with long experience on the frontline usually have much less confidence or enthusiasm for these demotic initiatives. The nature and delivery of our complex human activities are often very protean. Such formulaic systems of presentation and packaging, however well-intentioned, will serve them poorly.

Solutions? There are none. We can offer only our wisest compromises. In the past, I think we understood this better.

Ω

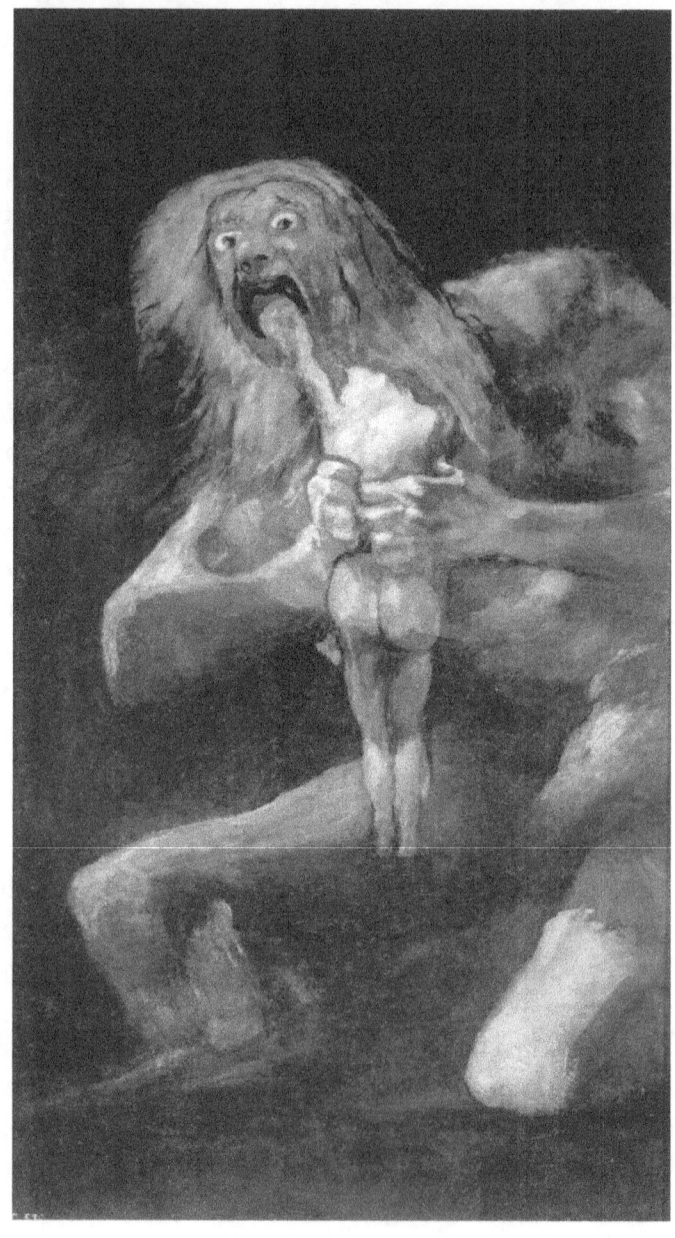

Francisco de Goya *Saturn Eating his Children*
1819 - 23

Institutional Atrocities

The malign vacuum from industrialised healthcare

Flagrant neglect or abuse in our care of the vulnerable within our advanced Welfare State seems shockingly perverse. How and why does this happen? This article argues that excessive industrialisation and schematisation are speciously alluring, but then alienating. Restitution of any culture of more compassionate care is like an organic process: it must develop from milieux that have receptive space for attachment, affections, and containment.

So, from the tide of depersonalised healthcare we have netted a flagrant and demonic example of maleficent neglect at Mid Staffs and, now alarmed, subject it to forensic analysis. Understandably we want to know: how could this happen? Who is responsible? Who can we blame? Government? Inspectors? Policymakers? Regulators? Practitioners? Administrative Managers? Clinical Managers? Almost immediately we have rhetorical cries for justice and resolution: More trainings, inspections, management! Professional eliminations! Clear and strong leadership! Show-trials for public pillory!

All of these responses have relevance or truth yet seem, to me, to miss some deeper understandings about how advancing technology is changing not just our thinking, but also our configurations of human connection. Like our banking and economic systems, our problems extend far before and beyond our crises, or our judgements of villainy or technical incompetence. These events are grotesque aspects of Zeitgeist: we are all in this together. We are all easily, unwittingly, victims or perpetrators; we have much to understand.

In my exploration I have come to some different, though contiguous, ideas. At their centre is this: that healthcare has become too beholden to the objective, technical, systemic and informatic; that the unmindful excesses of these have driven out interpersonal understanding, attachment and, thus, instinctive and gratifying caring. We have ignored – at great cost – an omnipresent paradox in our care of others: that is, impersonal treatments and formulations (science) tend to countervailance with personal engagements and holistic understandings (art). Our contemporary healthcare thus requires a vigilant balance: to offer our best skill, effectiveness and humanity, we must be able to combine these opposing principles – to weave and titrate them – differently with each encounter.

Four decades ago I was mentored by doctors who, generally, had a canny awareness of the importance of such complex balances. Successive generations have lost this sentience in our cultural rush and thrall to the impersonally managed, measured and procedural. In our increasingly push-buttoned world we are increasingly uncomprehending or intolerant of anything else.

I recently watched a BBC Newsnight programme: graphic descriptions of cowered, helpless people dying of dehydration on soiled sheets exampled our problems. The fractious lobbyists and pundits exchanged recriminations and accusations and never-again contritions. Several talked of inadequate or incorrect training, assuming that it is training that prevents a gravitational drift to blatant inhumanity. My view is different. Such omissions of care and connection are not a matter for adding specialist training, but of retaining or reclaiming our common humanity. How have we lost this, and on such a massive scale? How do we repair this, and in a way that will be sustainable?

In answering these questions it is important that we first acknowledge the blessings from our accelerated industrialisation of healthcare, for these have certainly brought us dramatic benefits alongside the insidious losses we are exploring here. The benefits are greatest for complaints that are primarily physically localised, and then are speedily and decisively resolved by procedural expertise. Clear examples are timely interventions in cardiovascular disease and some cancers. The way we systemise deliveries of such blessed interventions can be thought of as being like a factory.

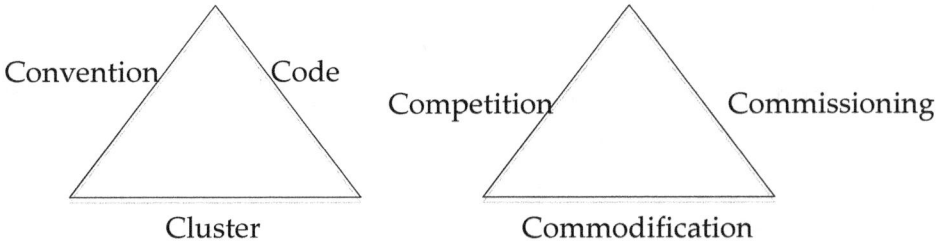

Figure 1:
Generic ordering of structural illnesses

Easy to measure and subject to 'factory' processes

Impersonal

Figure 2:
The current boost of industrialised healthcare

Designed to optimise management, measurement and 'factory' efficiencies

Impersonal

Yet the modelling of healthcare solely on this illness/procedural intervention paradigm is hazardous: when our suffering or its causes are not easily despatched, we need a culture that encourages something very different –attachments, affections and containments that develop between people. This enables personally anchored understanding and care: these offer not only comfort, but also the subtle inductions of healing within the person: of immunity, growth and repair. These activities cannot be schematic, but they are vital and vitalising. Notably attachments, affections and containments are at the heart of any healthy kind of family.

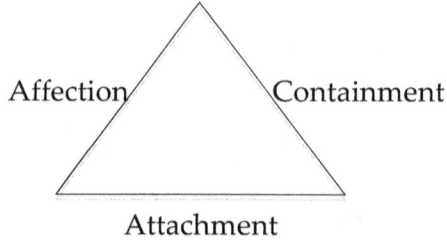

Attachment

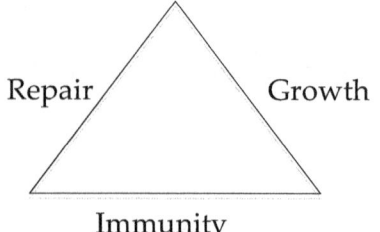

Immunity

Figure 3:
Interpersonal healing inductions

The 'family' ethos of well-fared welfare

Difficult to measure

Personal

Figure 4:
Intrapersonal healing inductions

The 'family' effects of well-fared welfare

Difficult to measure
Personal

While factory and family healthcare paradigms both have irreplaceable functions, their coexistence is not straightforward: for our best benefit can come only from ceaseless and careful choreography between them. Failure to understand, respect and achieve this delicate balance leads not just to ineffectiveness, but then to inhumanity or hazard. This is our current nemesis: our healthcare has become factory-rich but family-poor; informatics and scanner-sighted, but humankind-blind.

We have erred through our indiscriminate and thus excessive use of systematics: objectification, coding, planning and atomisation into managerially proliferated and boundaried specialisms. This may be a good way to run a robotic factory; it is definitely not a good way to raise a (healthcare) family.

Many will regard the Mid Staffs' debacle as criminal; I think it is more true, and more instructive, to think of it as cultural – Mid Staffs is thus a severe symptom, a warning sign, of our collective and collected errors. It is, of course, a severe event, but also one of many and now everyday examples of our healthcare anomie and human disconnection. This has happened both despite, and because of, our ever-increasing welter of commissioners, statutory bodies, dividing and divisive specialisms and competing autarkic Trusts – all these have led to a kind of healthcare that may look good as an architectural model, but is not good to live in. The worse the economy, the more impressive the economists.

I used to work in a much more heterogeneous NHS: the worse was worse, and the better much better. What was that 'better'? For the professionals working hours were longer, but morale was higher. Official Regulation was less, but vocational conscientiousness greater. Physical treatments were simpler and cruder, but personal care more sustained and sensitive. Electronic signalling non-existent, but conversational dialogue much easier. The pay was less, but the human reward was more. Didactic training facilities were meagre, but educational discourse richer. Most of my older mentors passed on loving care for their work, now my younger colleagues attempt to control others by formalistic Personal Development Plans.

And what of the patients? In the earlier, less technocratic NHS the better clinicians understood the importance of attachment, affection and containment in healing: we assured time, flexibility and imaginative space for these. We knew that such subtle interactions were often our best offerings of care for those conditions not easily cured – probably the larger part of our healthcare (yes!): our ageing, our mental distress, our tangled, troubled reactions to life's vicissitudes. For these our best efforts are more imaginatively pastoral than procedurally technical. Here the professional's integrity and judgement need personal enlightenment and nourishment, yet these are now often driven out by further technical management and training. The stark inhumanity at Mid Staffs is what happens if we do not understand and then neglect this delicate ethos of human connection; it is not about the kind of competencies that can be quickly and easily trained and regulated. The realisation of this may be an awakening, to reopen our eyes, hearts and minds.

This schematic desiccation of human connection in NHS healthcare is thus seminal to many of our serious and widespread problems. Over the decades I have observed this previously humanity-rich but imperfect organisation become more and more machine-like. People in the NHS I now work in, have a steadily declining personal knowledge or understanding of one another. In this ex-human vacuum the computer now sits, like a glowering, increasingly obese and enthroned emperor, appropriating the impersonal hub and frontline of administrative and informatic continuity.

What does this lead to? Anomie and depersonalisation. Few people can now name their GP, hospital consultant, or even the name of the specialist clinic they attend – mostly the computer will bid and book them, and mostly they will comply. GPs are increasingly working in large conglomerate practices where they offer little personal continuity of care, do not know families, neighbourhoods or even the names of their own receptionists. The receptionists, in turn, are disconnected from their (many) doctors and increasingly from the patients – 'reception' is now often done by a computer screen, leaving the receptionist 'free' to tend the computer with other tasks. Those other tasks often involve some kind of electronic data-collation, which will be necessary for the doctor to have on the screen, when he is having a procedural (non) contact with a patient he will never really get to know, and does not look at (because he is instead looking at the computer screen) … Get it?

In hospitals this anomic haze is even worse. In my local airport-like hospital I have seen consultants doing ward-rounds with rota-directed junior doctors they have never met before, attended by nurses who do not know their own colleagues, the patients or any other ward staff. This consultant, clustered with strangers, then attempts quickly to evaluate a complex (for we are) human/technical problem in a patient he is seeing for a first and (often) only time. Such a symphony of fragmented depersonalisations has been orchestrated by successive layers of 'improvements' to logistics and efficiencies of healthcare's training, standardisation, procurement and delivery. Examples? Amalgamation of medical schools, the dispersal of hospital nursing schools to universities, standardised modular trainings (rather than apprenticeship-type education), the encouragement of subcontraction, the abolition of GP personal lists, autarkic powers of NHS Trusts, payment by results, the fragmentation of 'Psychological and Psychiatric Care' into complex speciality-based streams, the European Working Time Directive, and, of course, the 3 'Cs' (Commissioning, Competition and Commodification) … all of these exampled initiatives – plotted and hatched by experts – have added to the remote-control complexity of our healthcare machine and the human inaccessibility for its operators and operatees.

*

Authentic caring is not a commodity to be traded or a skill-set to be instructed. It is an ethos, a metaphorical effusion of the heart. It is a benign, often relayed, human transmission that tends to mirror, then amplify, the incoming signal. It is a similar, but opposite, process to the contagious relay of cruelty, bullying or intimidation. For caring we need holistic imagination – to perceive or conceive more than is explicit or apparent. In contrast, cruelty requires us to see in a person or situation less than is clearly there. Cruelty is a kind of reductionism. Yet out current systems of management will urge us to the simplistic, formulaic and formalistic. Trust-employed healthdroids are now paid to look only at one prescribed part of complex problems, and in the Trust's officially prescribed manner. This is usually influenced significantly by the Trust's interests of autarky or economy.

Caring for others also depends on our own morale: whether we feel cared for, embraced by human connection and value. This, of course, will depend much upon our milieu: as health carers how do we perceive our working and employing culture? What kind of 'factory' or 'family' do these represent for us, and in what kind of ratios?

The quality of how we care about our care of others depends on ensuring receptive and imaginative mental space and time to make possible personal attachments. From these may develop affections: the investment of bonds with discernable feelings – for now we become significant, then important, for one another. This establishment of affectionate attachments then makes possible another and essential aspect of compassionate care: containment – we bring comfort, calm and often understanding to others when we receive, hold and share what they can no longer bear alone. Again, this is often a relay effect: the sufferer is helped to contain their suffering by feeling contained by the helper, who can do this much more readily if he himself feels an equivalent caring containment in his environment. Caring containment is thus passed on in successive relationships, like Russian Dolls, one within the other. It is important, so reiterated, that the opposite experiences and effects – of indifference, fear, cruelty etc – are passed on in a similar way. Thence come our dysfunctional or hostile families and institutions. Was Mid Staffs such an example of discontainment?

So, caring and containment can be best assured where attachment and affection can develop. As we have seen, this is unlikely in an NHS in which the ethos of the 'factory' has largely driven out the 'family'. Consider, for example, an undramatic and very common scenario: the process of a hip replacement in 1983 and again in the more industrialised/ schematised 2013.

1983. A technical task: personal continuity

Ali is 65-years-old and already crippled and housebound by his hip arthritis. He goes to see Mr O, an orthopaedic surgeon. Mr O hears Ali's story and complaint: Ali tells Mr O of how his life has been diminished and disempowered by his infirmity. Mr O recommends a standard hip replacement and sees Ali several times before and soon after the successful procedure, and then for longer-term follow up. The two men develop a low-key but cordial and discernable affection. Ali expresses his gratitude for a much restored life and feels encouraged by Mr O's interest and advice early in his recovery: he talks of him warmly as 'my surgeon' – this is affectionate, not presumptuous or possessive. Mr O is grateful, too. It is good for him to see the human effects of his technical intervention, to hear from Ali about a life restored. Mr O's work is often difficult and stressful: such human contacts nourish and sustain him, too. One of his young and idealistic students once tried to interest him in a conversation about Holistic Medicine. Mr O had replied that he'd never really understood what the term means; he was 'just a surgeon'. For Ali he was more: Mr O knew this, but did not speak of it.

2013. A technical task: a production line

Ali is Ali's son: he, too, has succumbed to a similar disability at a similar age. Ali attends the same hospital as his father had, but its inner workings are now very different and Mr O has long retired. There seems to Ali no equivalent or replacement for his father's surgeon, for he sees someone different each time he goes to the hospital. He does not know if the stranger he is talking to is a nurse, a doctor or a physiotherapist and he does not feel he should ask. Nor does he remember the names of the different clinics, but takes the appointment letter with him to ensure his accurate destination. He is seen by different practitioners for orthopaedic assessment, preoperative assessment, surgical admission, surgery, surgical recovery, and post-surgical follow up. He does not know the name of any of his attending clinicians or who replaced his hip. Ali thinks his technical care was 'probably alright', but confusing. He was afraid in hospital, but told no one. He found recovery painful, lonely and difficult: he had no quietly affectionate professional relationships to encourage him, and no smile of gratitude to bestow. 'Job done', true enough, but no human connection or deeper satisfactions for Ali or the anonymous 'Teams'. And the innominate, unknown hip surgeon – Mr or Ms O2 – what sustains them? What gives their tiring job human value and meaning?

*

Vernacular maxims: no statistics

After more than four decades as a frontline NHS Doctor I have mounting sadness and fear for the human and philosophical impoverishment of my profession. If I live long enough I, too, will have a serious role as a patient. The Mid Staffs exposure may shock many: for me it is merely another shard of disheartenment. Every working day I encounter similar, if lesser, systemic human disconnections. I look back over the rolling eras of errors, and management ideologies, and the hundreds of collegial conversations I had trying to make sense of them. In all of these I am searching for general caveats and motivational principles – the kind that might better guide institutions to enable, rather than stifle, imaginatively compassionate healthcare. Like the work itself, my compilation is flawed, never complete, and must always be revised:

- If we like our work and find it interesting, we will do it well and willingly.
- Such liking and interest often involves the gratification of seeing our work's longer-term evolution and personal effects. Deeper satisfactions, too, are often personal and holistic: conversely, fragmented, short-term work offers little of these.
- Encouragement to draw on our experience to make intelligent creative decisions is likely to engage and develop our best qualities. Submitting to endless committee-designated diktats does not.
- We thus prefer flexible and collaborative working arrangements rather than those that are rigid, competitive and divisive.
- If we get know people well, we will be well-motivated to care for them. The more you see of someone, the more of someone you see.
- If we do not know people it is far easier not to care, or even to collude with harm: History has innumerable examples prior to Mid Staffs.
- People who feel attached, interested and positively personally engaged need relatively little disciplinary or motivational management.
- In contrast, it is very difficult to get good work from people who do not enjoy their work, feel attached or positively, personally engaged: these are primary deficits, and no amount of regulation, management, training or financial incentive will rectify them.

Figure 5: *Imaginatively compassionate healthcare –*
some guiding caveats and principles

If large organisations, like individuals, can have breakdowns of spiritual and emotional integrity, then the NHS is set for an epidemic. This is largely due to our disinvestment of natural and positive attachments. Mid Staffs is but one early, now publicly flaunted, casualty.

*

The whole is more than, and different from, the sum of its parts.

Healthcare is a humanity guided by science.

That humanity is an art and an ethos.

Ω

Published in: *Journal of Holistic Healthcare*, Vol 10, Issue 1, Spring 2013

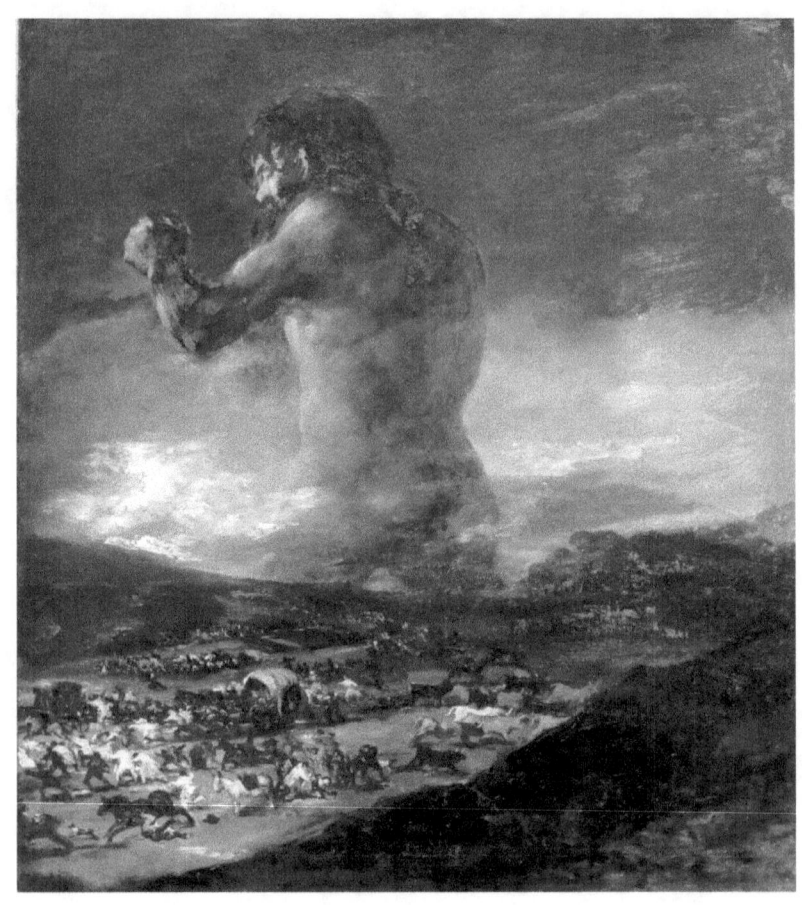

Francisco de Goya *El Coloso* 1808-1812

Beyond Orwell

Healthcare's hollow governance

Our smallest difficulties with others are often rich in political complexity. What does this mean? Two apparently trivial examples from healthcare administration are explored.

'Totalitarianism spells simplification: an enormous reduction in the variety of aims, motives, interests, human types, and, above all, in the categories and units of power.'

Eric Hoffer, *The Ordeal of Change* (1962)

'Men reform a thing by removing the reality from it, and then do not know what to do with the unreality that is left.'

GK Chesterton, *Generally Speaking* (1928)

Prologue: Brave New World

My formative years working in healthcare occupied a kind of pre-industrial world. The now ubiquitous and centre-staged rhetorics – to measure and manage – were then minor, quieter players. Like all industrialisations the transition has brought gains through losses: technical treatments are better, but personal care often worse.[1] The most parlous practitioners are now detected and removed earlier; but the pre-emptive management required to do this is often at the cost of our finer personal vocational identifications, devotions and initiatives: these often ail and then perish.[2] Healthcarers' technical errors may be less, but so too is vernacular human understanding. In forging such industry, we change the culture: a vocationally conscientious 'family' of practitioners has been steadily replaced by a 'factory' of centrally programmed and managed personnel: healthdroids.[3] A new term has been invoked to legitimise all this: governance.

The official intentions are sloganned into allures of healthcare improvements and entitlements to be delivered by ratchets of efficiency, equity and vigilant policing. [4]Increasingly these are procured and corralled by computer-compatible – thus electronically mediated and standardised – forms of surveillance and control.[5] While all this may work well with simpler tasks and scenarios, it elsewhere leads to perverse incentives and squandered resources.[5] Alarmingly, such

257

surveillance and control then develops hermetic and ineluctable qualities: no-one claims ownership or the authority to intelligently divert or discriminate.[6] Matters of subtle and sensitive welfare become rapidly and automatically delegated to new kinds of cybernated servomechanisms.[3,7] The complex galaxy of human needs and meanings must now submit to a culture of computer-templated compliance solely beholden to its own consistency and completion: a Frankenstein's Monster of non-humankindness, Technototalitarianism.[8] The following two apparently prosaic examples from General Practice are commonly endured though resented; rarely (as here) explicitly disclosed or discussed.

*

1. 'We've all got to do it. We've got to feed The Beast: that's the way we get the money.'

Eddie's distress is raw and naked: it is stark and disturbing and needs no further evidence for Dr T to know that Eddie needs much compassionate containment and guidance. Eddie's wounded sensibilities far exceed his meagrely educated capacities for articulation. His tremulous tearfulness bespeaks awakened shock from the past. This has conflagrated a subterranean arsenal of long 'forgotten' childhood memories: a leaden legacy that, til now, has wordlessly crippled his life. The force of this awakening has blown aside his frail defences: Eddie is now unable to stem the erupting intensity. His sense of fear, shame, humiliation and sorrow has accelerated beyond his words. Now, with Dr T he struggles to have a personally disclosing conversation for the first time in his life: his vocabulary is sparsely stocked. The doctor knows he must pay careful attention to these highly-charged but inchoate utterances. He will need his imagination, too, if he is to make much personal and systematic sense of this cloistered, encoded and intense drama. If he has any success Dr T will need much other help in his efforts to help Eddie: he starts the necessary contacts.

*

Eddie's first contact from the Psychology Service brings him bewilderment and alarm: he receives through the post a densely packed envelope. In it, amongst the legally required (but rarely requested) information documents and leaflets, there are many questionnaires. These firstly ask for wide-ranging personal and demographic details, and then there are those asking for more precise disclosure of the nature of his 'complaint'; its history and the severity of his disability. None of these make any sense to Eddie, who has needed all his courage to trust his few and difficult words with Dr T. He left school at 13: he is semi-literate. His level of distraction and distress make impossible the process of self-objectification required to competently complete such forms. More inadvertent though meaningful complexity emerges, for exposure to the questionnaire has itself worsened Eddie's fear of inadequacy and rejection: the 'science' pre-requisited as essential for the therapy has itself become countertherapeutic (and can offer only a contaminated vagary of science).

*

Dr T wants to procure psychological help for Eddie, yet he must also protect him from such procedural thickets he finds impassable. Dr T doubts that these complex routines will bring to Eddie any timely benefit. Yet to get this fragile man Diplomatic Immunity from the Psychology Department's Informatics Scanner is proving difficult. Dr T starts an escalade with their office staff and then Manager: their responses are polite but tethered – they have their instructions to instruct others. No, they are sorry they cannot accept exceptions. Next he tries a Senior Practitioner, SP, who baulks at what she considers Dr T's presumptive 'diagnosis' of Eddie. She attempts to explain to Dr T that 'psychological treatments' are now much more scientifically based and accurate: for Eddie to receive the benefits from these it is necessary for him to submit to these procedures – it is for his own good. Dr T wishes to demur and dissect, but SP instead wants him to submit to instruction, correction and compliance. He diplomatically disengages: he will try to recruit higher powers.

The Clinical Director, CD, another older practitioner, listens carefully to Dr T, who is relieved by CD's sanguine manner and open intelligence. His interest in people and their complexity seems still fresh and compassionate, but he now talks with a tired, stoic cynicism of the larger picture, of the vast, increasingly industrial NHS service to whose upper ranks he has been promoted.

CD is looking at a pencil which he taps on a note-pad, a discrete becalming rhythm, as if slowly Morse-Coding to unseen sympathisers. He raises his gaze to Dr T and smiles, a mixture of vicarious apology and conspiratorial sentience. His sigh is emphatic, a wished-for exhalation of greater difficulties.

'Yes, you and I both know how obstructive and redundant all this is, but it's the way we've got to do it. The way the System works now requires us all to produce the right data and statistics for our managers and Commissioners. We've all got to do it: we've all got to feed The Beast, otherwise the money doesn't come through and we don't get fed …'

*

2. 'Don't ask questions: just do it!
That way they make it easy for you.'

The week is a hard one for Dr T and his defence of any autonomous or vocational homeland: he is due for an Annual Appraisal, his ritualised submission to governance. This year it is with a much younger colleague, Dr YC.

Dr T's difficulties are mounting. For as successive appraisals have increased their demand for rigid format, formality and itemised detail, so has Dr T's difficulty in conforming to them. He is increasingly aware that the committee-consensused mindset and ethos come from a very different world of values and intent to his own. For decades he has been sustained by warmth and nourishment in his work, by a culture of unengineered and yet (mostly) mutually affectionate and respectful contacts with staff and patients. By assuming the primacy of such quiet attachments, other things have followed naturally: keeping curiosity and engagement fresh and alive; learning by his own enquiry, rather than others' protocol. His understanding of people, too, has been kept vernacular and fluid: he has avoided the crystalline solids, the public convenience-packs of devitalised psychiatric and social diagnoses. Essential to maintaining this engaged stamina is an enjoyment and wonder of our shared – yet often denied – human complexity – of ambiguity, paradox and semiotics. For behind the evident almost everything is also about something else. What? When is that useful? Who decides? How?

Dr T likes such questions, not for any clear or definitive answers, but because the process of questioning suffuses his mind and work with interest, light and life. If people become personally interesting they are much more rewarding to care for. Such questions have thus helped him start each of his thousands of working days with alertness, imagination and curiosity: for alongside our commonalities each moment, each individual, each encounter is unique. Such is the Art of Medicine.

But the new culture of governance, and thus its many employees, are now increasingly if unmindfully countervailed to such philosophy and holism, such semiotics and humanism. The language and format has consolidated as a commonality of schedules, items, boundaries, lists, measurements and prescribed plans.

*

Dr YC has a friendly manner and face. Her handshake is warm and reciprocal. Dr T is encouraged, but also wary of a brisk convergence in her movements and speech: she is a multi-tasking young woman and Dr T senses her bristle with delay.

Her survey of the voluminous obligatory documentation is more to identify anomalies and deficiencies than to pursue creative enquiry. She asks why Dr T has not filled out the section on his Professional Development Plan more fully and cogently. Dr T replies that he cannot: in more than forty years of exemplary medical practice and senior academic work, he has achieved a great deal, but has never had a private or public plan for any of it. His record has clearly been long, fertile and excellent, but never had governance. Dr YC draws in a breath and offers a brief mock-puzzled smile: 'Yes, I can see that – but it's not what is required now...'

Dr YC finds another failure: the selected Audit Project is not up to date: the Practice's documented and templated analysis of a defined area of prescribing is last year's. Dr T had not even been aware of his bureaucratic lapse. He is frustrated by being technically compromised about something that, beyond administrative formality, has little other value or meaning. What do they learn about him from such an audit? That he can think clearly? Can collect, collate and analyse data? That he can organise his staff? That he is mindful about prescribing? Surely, Dr T is surrounded by evidence that he can do all of these things. He also knows that such ubiquitously harvested audits are hardly read by anyone: they are perused and inspected, to see only if they pass muster. Usually they are then quickly cybertised for an oblivious eternity. Why, then, are thousands of doctors, throughout the land, having to spend time on projects that have no evident benefit or interest to anyone?

Dr T has a view: that such requirements of governance are rituals of hegemony, demonstrations of roles of dominance and submission, and shibboleths of acquiescence. They indicate – in diplomatic code – who is in control and who will obey, who is the definer and who the defined, who decides language and meaning. It also implies the spectre of professional extinction for non-conformists. Like an electric-fence for cattle, it may itself have flimsy structure, but its sharp, hidden signals quieten and control vast populations.

Dr T thinks this cattling of professionals raises important matters of integrity: not just his own, for he has seen the effects throughout the Welfare Services. He tries to interest Dr YC, but her cordiality is timed-out and is evaporating to irritated fluster:

'You may be right, but I have two children I must soon collect from school: I simply don't have time to talk about that kind of thing...'

She looks at her watch with tensioned resolve, and then toward Dr T, as if throwing him a line:

'Look ... a lot of us know that most of this is nonsense, but we've got to do it, so we do. My advice to you is: Make Things Easy For Yourself. Don't ask so many questions. Just do it! That way they make it easy for you...'

*

1984 in 2013: Epilogue in dystopia

Dr YC's brief attempt to rehabilitate Dr T awaits fruition and formal process. While his fate and intent remain doubtful he has an impulse to look again at George Orwell's 1984, a book he first read well before that date. Then the book was prophetic; now it occupies historic prophecy.

Dr T is unsure of the origin of his urge to return Back to The Future, but he thinks it is something to do with his encounters with CD and Dr YC. He thinks now of his early life, shadowed by relics and prophesies of totalitarian malignity. Bomb-wrecked, hollow buildings; shuddered, fresh fragments of tales of Samurai or Nazi atrocities; revered and mantle-pieced photographs of the keen-eyed, young deceased; silently or expletively despised images of the violently fallen, ogrous, totalitarian dictators – these picture his 1950's memories. That era gradually gave way to a quieter, more insidious, totalitarian menace: the Great Bear's Communism and the long Cold War. The fear and evidence of The Enemy at the Gate became less visible; the communal experience was less clear, more of an undertow. It was at this time that Dr T first read the, then, prophetic 1984.

As Dr T revisits Orwell's world, he notices his disparate reactions of gratitude and gloom. The harsher, barer aspects of Winston Smith's Oceania are mercifully absent: the endless war, the dreary physical deprivations, the mortal hazards of exposed dissent, the ubiquitous transmitted images of the nation's salvation and nemesis, of Big Brother and Goldstein.

But he has also ominous awareness of less flagrant similarities. He thinks of Oceania's omnipresent television screens and loudspeakers endlessly streaming public information, statistics and diktats, of the screens that spy as well as transmit. He thinks of Oceania's Doublethink: then thinks again of CD and Dr YC – how they must also fork their tongues to keep their jobs.

Dr T thinks of other subtle and geared-down similitudes. In the last decade he has seen his previously benignly-spirited, if sometimes heterogeneous, profession become drilled into a cowed, dispirited, orderly hive of healthdroids – of obedient supplicants or prescriptive commissars. True: there is no Room 101, yet Dr T has seen colleagues' fear – how anxious they are to show evidence of conformity: how their professional behaviour and speech then becomes a self-conscious, imitative, stilted carapace. There may be no party uniforms, yet such uniformity of thought, conduct and vocabulary have successfully completed their tasks: uniformed attire becomes unnecessary. Much of the conformity is anchored and assured by Technototalitarianism:[7] the now requisite pathways, algorithms, templates, key-words, codings and procedures. How and what to think or say is decided by unseen authorities. Thought and dialogue outside prescribed agendas, boxes or codes becomes increasingly irrelevant, uncomprehended and eventually subversive. Independence implies dissent; dissent is a precarious perch: there is unemployment beyond.

Dr T has glimpsed the faint, secreted, spectre of procrustean murders – the quiet expedience to remove any obstructions to the industrialisation of Welfare Services. He has seen the constructed and fatal undermining of well-respected and liked colleagues who failed to demonstrate timely enthusiastic alacrity for the new colonising trusts and plans. It is The Plan that must endure: individuals can be airbrushed from the picture. For the survivors, disquiet is quiet, murmured and brief – survivors have gratitude for their jobs. That gratitude turns fragile and nervous.

*

Dr T is talking to another senior survivor, Dr S. This sixty-year-old cohort may be assumed to be more secure and comfortable in this driven and industrialised culture, for he is a long-established advisor to government: a citizen in the citadel.

Dr T tells his old cohort first of his recent experiences and then of his tangled thoughts and feelings: he wants a thoughtful and experienced view from the other man, not quick and expedient commiseration or collusion. He is encouraged as Dr S seems intently attentive and sympathetic, nodding and softly ahaing. Dr T takes care, and whatever impartiality he can muster, to convey clearly his knotted frustrations.

He thus curbs his urge to overtalk and pauses, leaving a short, silent rest for his weltered thoughts. Dr S sits quietly too, as if in meditation, separating then gathering his thoughts. From this brief hiatus Dr S gazes and speaks. His directness has a soft, slow deliberation; he has clearly been incubating his thoughts well-prior to this encounter:

'Yes, I am of a similar inclination and generation to you, so I am sympathetic but, alas, not effectively so as I am beleaguered and outflanked by factors beyond my control or – and this is both alarming and deeply depressing – anyone's. Sometimes we introduce administrative or regulatory devices, believing they are sensible and helpful, only to find later that they are difficult to stop, and that their overgrowth has become more of a problem than the one we are trying to solve in the first place.

Sometimes the overgrowth spreads and roots rapidly: these devices, planted on the surface, leach into the subterraneum to produce culture; both our consciousness and unconsciousness change – we cannot easily rescind such things. We now live in a world that expects speed, standardisation, convenience and clearly labelled packaging. We've set that up in healthcare, and it's initially certainly brought us some advantages, but now we can't stop … so we continue to try to turn all healthcare problems into computer-compatible data, mass-produced processes and then a complex economic system that commodifies and trades in these. This speeding juggernaut is now difficult to brake: we now have hundreds of thousands of NHS staff whose salaries, status, homes – whose livelihoods, even identities – depend upon occupying a role in this healthcare emporium. And then the people who are likely to do best in all this are those most surrendered to the culture: those who most believe it…'

'So it's just like Orwell's 1984', says Dr T, offering what he tritely thinks is a pithy summation.

'Oh, no! This totalitarianism is much more refined – and probably durable – than our fictional 1984', Dr S quickly retorts, a slightly acerbic and ironic taint to a residually courteous manner. 'Our system doesn't need endless wars, flagrant scapegoats, monolithic and ever-present leaders or a life-threatening Secret Police: our system now largely runs itself: that's one definition of culture. There isn't really anyone in charge! Even at my level many of my colleagues seem – to me – unaware of how much they have bought into the package and thus speak the language. In my meetings with them I try to influence quietly: with patience, stealth and diplomacy. But I'm careful to stay in The Tent: if you're outside The Tent you have little influence, and you probably won't be heard…'

Dr T protests against his own agreement with this: his interruption intends reason, but is soured by concealed, petulant grievance:

'The problem with that is if you stay in The Tent long enough you lose your own voice and vision, and end up talking there like everyone else.'

Dr S sidesteps the beginnings of this angry charge, like a seasoned and taciturn matador:

'Well, in my case I hope that is incorrect. But I have more than myself to hold onto: my wife and family … my mortgage is not yet paid off, and I have two teenage children still to put through university…'

Dr T is quiet again, but differently, now gently melted with fresh and protective contrition.

All is not what it seems. Citadel? Yes. Citizen? Yes, but also hostage.

Dr T imagines a conversation he would like to have with George Orwell.

*

'*Everything begins as mystique and ends as politics.*'

Graffito, Wall in Paris, Student Protest, 1968

Ω

Language is not just Data

it is a custodian of our humanity

Computers and informatics have become central to NHS healthcare. All experience and activity are now subject to official technical designations. This changes our communications: language becomes increasingly lackeyed to the computer's requirements. Much else is lost. What?

'If language is not in accordance with the truth of things, affairs cannot be carried out to success.'

Confucius, *Analects* (6th century BC)

I suppose I was lucky, but then – at some level – I chose them, too. Beyond that, and more importantly, we were all part of a culture that could accommodate – even foster – such things. My first mentors in General Practice and Psychiatry – galvanised by the just departed 1960s – were all nourished, enlivened, then enlightened by literature and philosophy. Such proclivities were not ponderous or self-conscious postures, but pursuits that were shared with a mien of quiet and unaffected pleasure. I remember many conversations where, in order to understand others better, we made wefts of contemporary pragmatic practice with illuminated threads from drama, philosophy, literature or mythology.

The then-fresh Balint movement, too, encouraged us to step up and out from our scientific base of standard diagnoses and treatments; while we recognised that these certainly helped us, they could do so only with generalities. So grounded, we were spurred to thoughtful experiment: to engage with the humanly speculative and imaginative – for these could help us, instead, with the individual: this person and this situation. To do any of this we needed to draw from a panoply of human thought and testament. Imaginative understanding of others is a kind of 'play', and for any successful foray into play we must encourage an expanded, rather than constricted, language. For sometimes it is an unusual word, simile or metaphor that catalyses greater understanding and then rapport.

Even at the most pragmatic levels of service this previous broader and richer language was more likely to capture and convey the uncodifiable untidiness of real life, the crucial vicissitudes of Practice. I recently had an unexpected reminder of this, and it is a good example. While seeing Matthew, an amiably direct, stalwart and unnervously jocular thirty-five-year-old, I rummaged through his old manual records. I found there a mechanically-typed letter from a hospital Casualty Department. It was written to me in 1980 about a toddler, Matthew. Here it is:

"Dear Doctor
Matthew P, age 2 years

This delightful little boy was brought here on Sunday morning by his very anxious and solicitous mother. Mother was worried by an alleged fever and cough of two days' duration. Matthew himself was alert, bright-eyed, active and playful. He had no signs apart from a very mild catarrhal cough, which he didn't seem to notice!

Mother seems a sensible and intelligent woman, but inordinately anxious about Matthew's minor symptom. In talking to her it came to light that her own sister has recently been diagnosed with Acute Leukaemia. Understandably this has shocked and shaken the family. I had a long discussion with Mrs P in which I told her that Matthew is perfectly well apart from having a slight cold, and that her very real anxieties about her sister have unintentionally spilled over onto Matthew. I hope I have been able reassure her. I have taken the liberty of asking her to see you for follow-up.
Yours sincerely
Dr TS, CSO"

All these years later I remember a couple of phone conversations I had with Dr TS – a warm, friendly, bantering Northern voice that conveyed intelligent pleasure in his work, its people and their welfare. Reading this letter, more than thirty years later, brought me both joy and sorrow.

The joy was humble though clear; it was the memory of such quiet, subtle suffusions of personal interconnectedness: here Dr TS had shared with me his brief connection with – but growing understanding of – Matthew, Mrs P and all her family. Matthew's slight catarrhal cough was thus given much greater human – and thus healing – meaning. This sent a gentle benign ripple across the whole matrix: we all felt better about ourselves, one another and our work. This is well-fared welfare.

But then came my sorrow, for the massive yet little-voiced loss of such things. For it is almost impossible that I would receive such a letter now. Both because of, and in spite of, the endless blizzard of electronic, data-particled e-mails transmitted from my local airport-like hospital, I have with them almost no conversations enlarging my understanding of people. Dr TS's personally sentient letter would now be replaced by an anonymised electronic, templated format. This would machine-gun me didactically with tabulated impersonal data itemising myriad aspects of the (normal) physical examination; the healthy child's measurements of oximetry, temperature and respiratory rate; the immunisation status; the social status of the child and whether Social Services' involvement has been triggered … This surfeit of (usually) unedifying administrative detail would have neither space nor vocabulary for the brief glimpse of the importantly unobvious; the human story that gives this (non) medical scenario significant and compassionate meaning. We have lost both the personal language of healthcare and its collegial discourses.

Such losses coalesce, then anchor. Eventually a restricted language and format will not merely confine description, it will – hypnotically – limit our thinking and actions too. Language, thought and action are often less divisible than our analyses of them. Expansion or contraction, encouragement or proscription, nourishment or impoverishment – influence one and the others will probably change in a parallel way.

The more complex the human activity, the more this matters. We have seen, with Matthew, how language can service or disservice a relatively simple, yet humanly-complexed, medical problem. Let us take a more intricate and chronic problem. Geoff is a troubled dis-eased man in his mid-30s. Here are two accounts from an encounter he has with a psychiatrist.

A. Patient as object. Language as designation

G has a long history of agitated depressive illnesses with marked anxiety/panic components. Although his questionnaired depression scores were high, they were discrepant from the MDT staff's assessment. He has a poor record of maintaining work and long-term relationships. He also has problems with anger management: this was evident to the Clinic Staff when I was unavoidably delayed. This inconvenience was clearly explained to G, who nevertheless was unacceptably angry and rude to the staff in response. It is thus likely that G also has a Personality Disorder.

B. Patient as person. Language as understanding

G has never recovered from the childhood terror and sorrow from his experience of father's raging cruelty, brutality, and then final desertion. G's life has been spent yearning for, but mistrusting, male support, esteem, affection and affiliation. He wants comfort from others, but fears betrayal, so disguises his needs. My lateness for his appointment seems to stir in him ancient residues of imperilled dependency, uncertainly and abandonment. His response to my greeting is staccato, flushed and tense: he seems both angry and afraid. I sense in him a conflation of fight and flight, and I think again of his wounded, early childhood.

*

If it were you that was distressed, which doctor would you wish to tend you?

*

One definition of the success of a Specialty is that it replaces vernacular language with its own vocabulary. Thus specialisation both colonises and short-circuits common speech, replacing this with its own distillate. The losses involved vary greatly: the dehumanising potential of 'Megaloblastic Anaemia' is negligible, that of 'Depression' considerable.

Archimedes' notion of displacement is instructive far beyond the physical world: it often operates in the realms of human culture and language. The overgrowth of the technical and the schematic can all too easily – without malign design – extinguish the organic and the human. Our world of ever-increasing mass-production has many hidden taxes. There are hungry conundrae, too: how do we safeguard literature in our language, art in our (medical) science and heart in our practice?

*

'A man is hid under his tongue'

Ali Ibn-Ali-Tabib, *Sentences*, (7th century)

Ω

Published in *British Journal of General Practice*, March 2014

Post Mid Staffs:

A Plenitude of Platitudes

Mid Staffs refers to the Mid Staffordshire NHS Trust in the UK, which has been clearly exposed, in numerous cases, of flagrant and gross neglect of care of vulnerable, usually elderly, hospital in-patients. Many of the examples far exceeded privation or indifference of care, and had qualities of active cruelty, even sadism. There is much further evidence that such abuse is widespread throughout the UK NHS, though Mid Staffs may be an extreme example. While individual responsibility must always be important, the Mid Staffs debacle has raised gravely important questions about the nature, direction and ethos of UK NHS healthcare culture.

Can the harmful excesses of depersonalisation in healthcare be usefully addressed by further redesign of systems and management? Or do we need a different kind of thinking and vocabulary?

The worse the economy, the better the economists.

Likewise, Post Mid Staffs, we are now blessed with a tranche of experts who talk confidently of management designs that can lead us quickly to the clear, Sunlit Uplands of healthcare.

In the last week[1] we have heard, for example, from Nick Seddon,[2] Geoffrey Robinson[3] and Lord Ara Darzi.[4] All talk in a similar revelatory manner from a common stock of maxims and metaphors. Here are some: 'Greater transparency', 'opening up the cutting edge of practices', 'celebrating and rewarding success; identifying and rooting out underperformance', 'turbo-boosting quality', 'putting measurement at the heart of safety culture', 'improving workforce by enforcing links between pay and performance', 'zero tolerance of failure', 'centralised systems of reporting and review': all these sound-bitten imperatives are late seedlings of Jeremy Bentham's Prisons' *Panopticon*[5] and BF Skinner's behavioural carrots and sticks. This history of attempts to systemise and control human behaviour is instructive: limitations are evident.

What these pundits seem not to consider are the aspects of caring that involve ethos and vocation: imaginative empathy and compassionate attachment. Their offerings seem devoid of

---

[1] The week beginning 18/2/13. The quotes are taken from newspaper articles and media interviews of that week.

[2] Nick Seddon. Deputy director of Reform, an independent think-tank.

[3] Geoffrey Robinson. Businessman, management guru and TV presenter.

[4] Lord Ara Darzi, chair of the Institute of Global Health Innovation, Imperial College, London. Previously a Minister of Health.

[5] Jeremy Bentham (1748-1832) was a philosopher, jurist and social reformer. His Panopticon was a design for prisons, enabling the jailers to have constant view of all their prisoners.

any philosophy of pathos or ethos: how and why should we care for one another? What motivates altruistic transcendence?

It is such psycho-spiritual considerations that seem, to me, glaringly absent from the current debate and – most importantly – from the system we have created – the culture that then creates such dissociated, alienated atrocities in healthcare. Perversely, our pundits then offer us yet more depersonalised thinking to counter depersonalisation.

For all its more primitive technology and heterogonous management, I found my previous decades of work in NHS healthcare far more personally imaginative, responsive and respectful.

In our impatient quest for Welfare Services efficiencies, we have compressed our welfare to behave like object-spewing factories. Such industrialisation has expediently jettisoned our human attachments, connections and understandings. Offered here is an alternative assortment of maxims that can help us re-route our culture, so that we may re-root our humanity in healthcare:

Imaginatively compassionate healthcare
– some guiding caveats and principles

• If we like our work and find it interesting, we will do it well and willingly.
• Such liking and interest often involves the gratification of seeing our work's longer-term evolution and personal effects. Deeper satisfactions, too, are often personal and holistic: conversely, fragmented, short-term work offers little of these.
• Encouragement to draw on our experience to make intelligent creative decisions is likely to engage and develop our best qualities. Submitting to endless committee-designated diktats does not.

- We thus prefer flexible and collaborative working arrangements rather than those that are rigid, competitive and divisive.
- If we get know people well, we will be well-motivated to care for them. The more you see of someone, the more of someone you see.
- If we do not know people it is far easier not to care, or even to collude with harm: History has innumerable examples prior to Mid Staffs.
- People who feel attached, interested and positively personally engaged need relatively little disciplinary or motivational management.
- In contrast, it is very difficult to get good work from people who do not enjoy their work, feel attached or positively, personally engaged: these are primary deficits, and no amount of regulation, management, training or financial incentive will rectify them.

Looking back, I can see that it is such notions that sustained and nourished my generation of better practitioners over long, gratifying and appreciated medical careers. Such ways of thinking of, and relating to, others used to grow naturally from certain kinds of culture and education. They fare far less well in our current forced march to homogenised and hegemonised management or trainings.

Sticks, carrots and panopticons are often poor motivators for the more complex aspects of human care.

*

Healthcare is a humanity guided by science. That humanity is an art and an ethos.

*

We must beware.

Ω

'GPs know their Patients, Families and Communities'

– Really?

GPs are increasingly employed as task-directed, upper-echelon *healthdroids*. They are losing the pastoral skills that depend on holistic views and vernacular understandings. Why is that?

During the first week of the new GP-led commissioned NHS, a televisioned young doctor offered this GP-led soundbite: 'GPs know their patients, families and communities.'

Really?

My experiences as a long-serving GP, and as a recently signed-up patient, are very different. Your GP is now likely to be part-time, short-term and serving in a multi-doctored practice where *personal* continuity is increasingly rare. You are thus likely to see a doctor you have never seen before, and when you see them they may see even less of you, as they will probably spend more time looking at the computer screen. Commuting to work, they are unlikely to have a personal home or roots in the immediate neighbourhood. They may develop some knowledge of one of your 'conditions', but almost none about your nature, story, family or life-milieu. They are most unlikely to know your kin. The better among the previous generation of 'Family Doctors' responded well to all of these. They mentored me; I witnessed this, just as I now see its disappearance.

There are many causes for this loss of more personal healthcare. Among some of the avoidable causes are: the managerial hostility to small practices (favouring large impersonal conglomerates), the abolition of Personal Lists (thus devolving the interested responsibility of a particular doctor to a large, generic 'Team'), the sub-contraction of Out of Hours services to agencies (that are unlikely to have any personal knowledge or bond at times of greatest vulnerability and need), the increasing use of shorter-term, sessional, commuting staff (who have no vernacular knowledge, roots or interest in the locality). How can doctors working in these conditions develop personal and holistic understandings of any length and depth?

Doctors are not unique in this disinheritance. *Postman Pat* used to be a reassuring hub of the community; a fount of local human and geographic knowledge. Alas, our postman now is often only recently employed, a new immigrant, and himself, lost and asking for directions…

Marketisation cannot buy or commission the kinds of bonds, understandings and communities that constitute the human heart of healthcare. But marketisation can destroy them.

Hello, Health Commissioner. Goodbye, Family Doctor?

The new healthcare reforms and their threat to personal doctoring

The idea, now diktat, that GPs should lead the complex provision of healthcare for localities may subtract more than it adds to overall health-welfare. How and why could this happen?

'Simplicity is the most deceitful mistress that ever betrayed man.'

Henry Adams, The Education of Henry Adams (1907)

Today, the first day of the new era of GP-led NHS commissioning, I saw a young GP on the television. She was interviewed to sample a voice of professional support and enthusiasm for the just-hatched, reformed regime. She spoke with an authoritatively quiet manner and an assured economy of phrase. She said: 'GPs know their patients, families and neighbourhoods.' A think-tank pundit, later in the programme, said much the same. Their views sounded solidly sincere, weighted with the calm dullness of uncontentious fact. On reflection, though, what I heard was specious – optimistic and plausible sounding, but substantially misleading: for GPs' personal knowledge of patients is increasingly short and shallow.

Yes, their assertion was once true, yet even then only selectively so: of the better and more vocational GPs, until about twenty years ago. I was mentored by that kind of doctor: they mostly served smaller (than now) practices, full-time, often for several decades. This combination of smallness of scale, ethos of vocation and length of time-span made much easier certain kinds of personal bonds and understanding: these were dyadic (the doctor and his patient), familial (the patient and their family) and vernacular (their particular world, beyond the family boundary). So, yes, it is true that those kinds of doctors and their patients, in that generation, could more easily develop an informal and often inexplicit understanding of one another. Certainly I witnessed many times how these could, with quiet and subtle patience, lead to gratifying and healing encounters. For about three decades these natural nexae of healthcare developed – were fuelled by and then created – a vigorous culture of person-centred discussion and literature. The Balint movement was a good example of the flowering of this and its subsequent neglect.

The dissolution of this humanly networked healthcare started, then accelerated, from the beginning of the 1990s – the time of the first substantial computerisation and attempts at (internal) marketisation. This rationalisation has had many effects that few had anticipated or intended.

What has this led to? To healthcare far more able with generic management than with personal connection and understanding. True, this is variable and most evident in large (as most now are) hospitals. It may be less true in General Practice, but still a serious and growing problem: doctors and patients are increasingly personally unknown to one another.

What does this look like? Often now, GPs do part-time, shorter-term work in ever-larger centres. These populous, busy conurbations are more like the milling milieux of a contemporary airport then the personal refuge of an erstwhile Family Doctor. In these large health centres doctors engage a world that has turned increasingly computercentric: in the waiting room in many surgeries the patient is not now greeted by a receptionist, but by electronic self-registration on a touch-screen. Then, in the characterless consulting room, the doctor is incrementally yoked to centrally-determined, computer-designated impersonal tasks and an endless incoming tide of e-mails: in this cybersurgery colleagues and other staff become more accessible to electronic signalling than natural conversation. This computercentric abstraction and anomie leaches to patients, too. Consultations often rapidly default to an administratively correct form of data-harvesting or officially despatched response. The patient's unique voice is not really heard, the unspoken not imagined, their face not remembered. The computer may provide images of the abstract that too easily replace other realities.

We now have little literature, or even talk, of the vagaries of *relationships* in medical practice: the very real and fertile, yet so-often-elusive, heart of our work: three decades ago such personal understandings were regarded as essential staples, or vital keys to therapeutic contact. But such notions cannot be easily measured, standardised or mass-produced: they have been bulldozed aside by notions that can. The result is an unstoppable data-blizzard, an errant sophistication that will often blind our view of people.

The infusion of commercial and industrial maxims into healthcare is thus wide-ranging but unequally obvious. The previous example considered the problems arising from abstracting complex human problems into formulaic forms of quantifiable data. This has become nearly universal and thus cultural: easily seen and expediently accepted. Other, more particular aspects, are more easily overlooked: the little recognised yet massively influential abolition of GP Personal Lists is a good example. This little-consulted measure – to ease administrative facility and tidiness – has been widely destructive of person-centred GP bonds. It has led to an anomie where doctors and patients increasingly become strangers to one another. We lose the myriad and humbly unique personal understandings and investments – and then the gratifications and therapeutic possibilities that can emerge from these. The system may look tidy, but people feel lost ... and it is not just the patients.

*

So it is a sparse but diminishing truth that most GPs 'know their patients, families and neighbourhoods'. The reality is starker and harder.

*

Yet more trouble awaits us. For the contentious suitability for GPs to *lead* the commissioning will become more knotted (and notted) as it evolves. In previous times GPs' personal knowledge of people and their networks made them a valuable resource to be *consulted* for planning and management: paradoxically this was then little used. Perversely, now that GPs' special sentience has almost been destroyed, these semi-blinded, administratively-weary GPs are now commanded to *manage* the planning and management. Whatever little attention and interest GPs are now able to pay to the personal aspects of care will be further displaced and eroded by these new managerial demands. For the more doctors' heads and diaries are crammed with meetings, e-mails, action-lists, data, agendae, pie-charts, flow-charts, deadlines and algorithms, the less creative and personal attention they can pay to the people who come to them (or themselves).

The GP who is caught in hostile and litigated negotiations about tendered tariffs for hip-replacement surgery is far less likely to perceive or understand the significance of the recent death of a cat to a childless, lonely, elderly widow whose husband died last year. Such is a typical scenario from the near-future. Care needs certain kinds of imaginative receptivity. The time and space for these are easily crowded out. How do we ensure that the Healthcare Commissioner does not finally asphyxiate the Family Doctor?

*

Healthcare is a humanity guided by science.

*

We must beware.

*

'Seek simplicity, but always mistrust it.'
Alfred North Whitehead (1861-1947)

Ω

Publ. by *BMJ Group Blogs*, 7/6/13

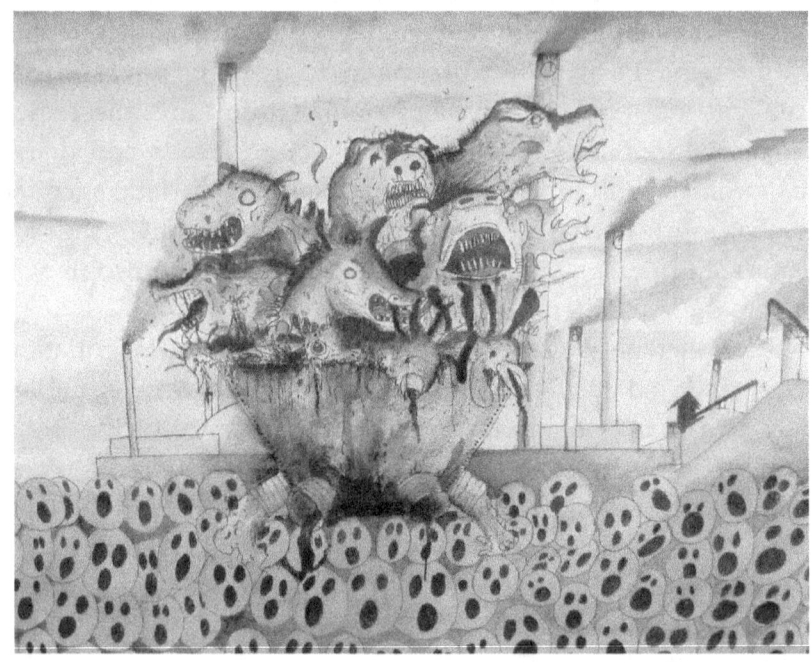

W. Hayemann – *Factory Farming*

Our Welfare is ill-fared by yet more strictures and structures

Surely, all Welfare professionals should forever be more strictly appraised and registered? Here are some reasons why not.

Tristram Hunt, Shadow Education Secretary, recently vaunted a policy to improve our state schools: that all teachers should be regularly and strictly appraised and licensed, as is now routine in the medical profession. This may seem overdue and briskly sensible. Yet wider experience shows that such plans and their consequences are often bewilderingly discrepant. This is a brief survey of that discrepancy.

We can probably all agree on our starting point: a wish for our Welfare professionals to have good personal, technical and ethical standards and skills. The crystallising rhetoric is always appealing and easy to construct. How to foster and assure these human qualities proves considerably trickier. What goes wrong, and why?

As a long-serving GP I have been increasingly witness and subject to this process: to managerially quality assure all NHS doctors. The results often turn paradoxically perverse: the laudable intent rapidly degrading into a bureaucratic maze of procedures, passable only by 'correct' statements of compliance. This rapid transition from aspirational to bureaucratic is now a common welfare anomaly and leaves a long wake of leaden consequences. For our consequent coagulations of acquiescence then obstruct the possibility of any more searching or authentic dialogue. Most doctors expediently practise recitation of the required protocols, shibboleths and submissions: this is called 'Preparing for an Appraisal'. The appraisal itself is usually undertowed and subtexted by compounds of fearful obedience, pragmatic stoicism or concealed resentment. In such a coercive charade how can anything real or useful be exchanged between practitioners and their governing bodies?

So, such formulaic attempts to govern welfare turn heavy, blunt and blind. Their success is restricted, possibly, to the most egregious or wilful failures of standards: the obvious ones. Our public safeguards have thus frequently relegated themselves to mere theatres of hegemony. This is an excellent current example of how, with good intent, substantial NHS time and resources are squandered. Goodwill is an early but lasting casualty.

Longer-term damage accrues insidiously: it is now wide and deep. For excessive and clumsy hegemony begets fearful compliance – and then the human terrain turns barren; our personal habitat becomes unable to nourish or sustain creative spirits of personal vocation and its gratifications. This is important because our best Welfare evolves from a delicate blend of self-responsible freedom and inner discipline. Clearly this kind of inner growth and balance cannot be simply conjured by yet more external rules.

Throughout Welfare our planners and politicians have lost sight of an important natural and human principle. It is this: people who like their work, generally, will want to do it well, and will need relatively little management. Conversely, those who do not like their work will be inveterately resistant to all management initiatives – be they payments, inducements, trainings, threats, goals, targets or deadlines. In Welfare particularly the nature of our human input cascades and amplifies: so, an increasing plethora of remote controls and formulaic edicts will produce demoralised and officious practitioners. Throughout education and pastoral healthcare, our positive influence comes more from attitude and morale than technical compliance and qualifications.

In NHS healthcare such principles are often disregarded in the stentorian 'driving up standards': the price we pay is akin to a stress-related internal haemorrhage. For example, we can readily adapt the imperative to eliminate the small number of severely substandard or rogue practitioners. But how do we do this without an even greater loss amongst the remainder: of morale, trust, goodwill and empathic vocation – the natural springs of professional humanity, collegial beneficence and thence good Welfare? For those doubting the seriousness of this question: look at the statistics about Welfare services workers –

these indicate clear and rapid rises in sickness, intrainstitutional litigation, career abandonment and early retirement. These are the human costs of disregarding such questions. Hence it is that the excess and heaviness of our management is ill faring our own welfare.

This wide range of evidence converges back to an observable truth that should now be a truism, but in our hustling business we have become heedless to. It thus merits reiterating: frustrated and etiolated Welfare professionals are unlikely to work well or to stay long. Our mounting healthcare debacles are yet another alarming reason for us to revisit and restore our investment in human connection and understanding – for this is the provenance of any wholesome realm of human care. These lessons may be currently sharpest in healthcare, but are seminal throughout our Welfare services.

To understand and nourish one another better in our indefatigably industrial world we must know when to take our hand off the ratchet and our foot off the accelerator.

Ω

Form Devouring Essence

When brokered services tend broken hearts

Our healthcare rhetoric of data and systems has largely destroyed our capacity to make the kind of personal bonds that understand and heal human dissonance. Stephen and his plight serve to illustrate and explore this.

1. A Prologuing Parable

'What would you like, Dali?' says Ali, from behind the Pizza Bar.
The Dalai Lama squints and marvels at the long list of offered combinations.
'I want One with Everything!' he replies, throwing his arms wide in rapture, to suggest Infinity.
Preparation takes Ali some time and the box is made up specially, the largest he has ever used.
To pay for it the Dalai Lama gives Ali the largest banknote he can procure and then waits, patiently at first.
'Can I have my change, Ali?' he asks eventually.
Ali sighs softly and shakes his lowered head slowly, with muted sorrow and disappointment: 'Oh! Dali! You, of all people, should know not to ask for this; that all Change must come from Within.'

The Tibetan Book of the Dudes 7th century BC, upgraded and rebranded version, 2014

2. Form devouring essence

Stephen's origins fifty years ago were chaotic and prophetic: an accidental conception by a young, brief and impulsive coupling. The unreceptive conceivers hurried to expediently jettison their conception: father rapidly for oblivion; mother bridled until Stephen's birth, then passing him to her own parents for care.

Stephen's early childhood was thus repaired and reprieved for a few, and the most, secure years of his life. Mother then met another partner and thought the omens were now right to start a more deliberate family. Through contention, then acrimony, then litigation between mother and her own parents, Stephen was removed from his grandparental loving home and returned to his parental and capricious source. Fate was not kind to any of the converged players in this new act: mother never had another live birth, and stepfather's geniality of promise turned to a sullen resentment of envious disappointment. The knot tightened and darkness gathered: indifference turned to sarcasm, slashing words conflated with beating fists and bodily shakings. Stephen shook, retroflected and planned escape. For her own security, mother colluded with power. Stephen left home age fifteen looking for some predictable and protective influence. He soon joined the Army.

Stephen never really found the peace or inclusion he craved. In his early adult life he lost himself in sports, macho banter, the consoling hazes of alcohol, drugs and thence to sexual deliria, with little-known partners. A brief marriage first absorbed such continuing assaults, then listed, capsized and sank, leaving a vengefully confused ex-wife adrift, huddling for comfort and buoyancy with their two sons. Stephen's growing awareness of how he was, in many ways, re-enacting his own abject beginnings was more than he could bear: he sought further escape through the only routes he knew – from the comforts that drew in his nemesis …

In his forties Stephen's life is slowing and he is beginning to see more clearly the pattern of his personal carnage. He tries to rebuild, but finds that this is akin to footholding sliding shale.

By his late forties his old defences are in terminal decline. His distress can no longer be distracted or buttressed and far exceeds his vocabulary. His signalling becomes urgent, intense, scrambled and uncontained. Dread, rage, guilt, fear, grief, shame, contrition all jostle to inhabit his confused and alienated loneliness. His offered quanta of anguish are inchoate and polymorphous: insomnia, panics, overwhelming physical symptoms – without – signs for the doctors, the sense that his mind and body are sometimes exploding and other times imploding and then colonised by others, consoling or persecuting superstition, bleak and suicidal despair, his fear of harming those that venture care or closeness: all are presented to A&E departments, Walk-In Centres, Out of Hours call centres, thence to Psychiatric Services and, finally, his new GP, me.

*

Stephen enters my room and my life for the first time seeming turbulent and adrift. I fine-tune the signals: I think I discern a mistrustful yearning for affection, inclusion and reassurance. An unbidden image fleets my mind: of a storm-tossed, mast-broken caique limping into the shelter of a small harbour. All of this is communicated to me wordlessly and will-lessly: I have intuition for his story – history – but this is not yet tethered by details. When disclosed, such details coalesce to warn of the difficulty of our task: we will need to offer Stephen several capacious and flexible containers – hearts, minds and diaries – to quieten, nourish, and heal him. Now, forty-five years after the disintegration of his brief exposure to wholesome family life, Stephen will need the best kind of family surrogacy our Welfare Services can muster. Such belated balm for his ancient wounds will not cure him, but slowly, from outside-in, it may awaken Faith, Hope and Charity* – *Agape* – the heart of healing.

*

Who will provide such supportive and guiding scaffolding? As his GP I can play a small yet important part, but I will need much help, particularly from psychiatric services. Yet here, where I am needing easy access to a bridge, I look out instead to a chasm: there is no 'family' to receive him, just a succession of placements.

To reify the metaphor: in one year Stephen was seen by many boundarised and separate Teams. Specifically: Hospital Liaison (3), Emergency Psychiatric, Home Treatment, In-patient, Community Mental Health for Mood Disturbance, Community Mental Health for Psychosis (his protean disturbance made distinctions only administratively meaningful), Psychology: Cognitive Behaviour Therapy, Psychology: Behaviour Activation Therapy.

Very significantly Stephen does not know the name of any of the Teams and cannot recall the names of any of their practitioners.

This anomie does not daunt the sharply missioned (now commissioned) Teams – for all, it seems, have an agenda to 'cure' him or, at least, to ensure brisk progress along a relayed 'Recovery Pathway'. This process, it seems, attempts to short-circuit more primal, powerful needs: these, through personal attachments, can create individual understanding and thence a growing, deepening capacity to create positive meaning and gratifying bonds.

Over many years an underlying principle – now increasingly disregarded – has become clear to me: that desired change comes often by an indirect route. Symptoms then dissolve not through direct countervailance, assault or ablation – what some like to confidently call 'management' – but by certain kinds of attuned and resonant apposition; the deliberate fostering and protection of certain kinds of *relationship*. Such constitute the inductions of *healing*, which contrast with the conductions of *treatment*. As a young psychiatrist in the 1970s I was engaged with many such personal projects. It was humbling and unglamourised work, but had quiet, slow, deep satisfactions. It was impossible to standardise and very difficult to measure, so we did not. This did not matter then because, in healthcare, we had not yet entered a world so tightly managed and systemised. The recently emergent healthcare realms have subsequently attempted to subsume all human problems and activities to standardised codes, procedures, quantifiable data and generically packaged Care Pathways. These ensure computer-compatibility, but there is a costly undertow: Technototalitarianism.

In my early years of practice the difficult work of looking after Stephens was much more possible: I had around me a collegial extended 'family' for synergy and support. Often these people got to know both the patient and myself, sometimes over many years; we developed a well-fared web of personal familiarity: welfare.

Such longer, personal, confluent contact has become almost extinct. My contact now is usually once-only with a sharply-boundaried, specifically-tasked duty-desk worker or Team Leader. Like Stephen, I feel my family has gone. My work has become homeless.

*

For the last decade, since the disintegration of my collegial family, I have been trying to understand the riddle of our increasing personal disconnection in healthcare. This is happening both in spite of, and because of, our mandates for 'efficiency': our increasingly resourced, ratcheted and managed systemisation. How and why have we created a culture that is less able to care for Stephen than forty years ago? What do we need to reclaim?

3. Re-anchoring essence

I think much can be explained by a little discussed, but seminally important, shift of axioms in planning, teaching and academia throughout pastoral and mental healthcare. We have abandoned the previous flexible equilibrium between *phenomenology* (a description and clustering of how things *are*, or appear) and *semiotics* (a speculation of what things might *mean*).

The significance of this needs a little elaboration. Phenomenology is more compatible with objective and scientific discourse and explanation. In contrast, semiotics is necessary for imaginative human understanding. So, phenomenology is more concerned with treatment, while healing must draw largely from semiotics. It is the thoughtful balance and dextrous exchange between the two that makes *holism* possible. The art of medical practice and compassionate care are mostly impossible without the broad, flexible intelligence of holism.

In the last dozen years there have been influences destructive to the fragile habitat of such holism. This is largely due to an accelerated coupling of computer use to projects aiming to standardise and industrialise all healthcare. This leads ineluctably to a reductionist healthcare rhetoric: to displace semiotics (an unmeasurable art) by phenomenology (in mental and pastoral health a proto-science, easily and speciously overdeveloped).

Such projects can readily turn to follies. Indiscriminate and overzealous attempts to forge a science of manipulation will risk extinguishing the art of understanding. This becomes much more likely as our NHS services are designed to be brokered – this is now implemented by such devices as autarkic and competing Trusts, Commodifying Commissioners, Payment by Results and competitive tendering. The consequent follies thus turn what should be artful science into a cult of *scientism*: hermetic systems of technical language and data which develop like monoculture farming and become inimical to wider questions and dialogue. Commercial and organisational interests almost always will be allured by such streamlined production and tamper-proof packaging. Hence form devours essence.

What we are losing are anchoring principles: *Healthcare is a humanity guided by science. That humanity is an art and an ethos.* How do we retrieve them? We must re-establish the more fragile art of healing alongside the now oligarchic science of treatment. We must create head and heart-space for the rich vicissitudes of human bonds and understandings. We must understand and respect the fact that the heart of many of our most precious experiences and activities cannot be directly codified and measured: they require conservation of different kinds of language and thought. When we have seriously understood these we might dare to take our hand off the ratchet and our foot off the accelerator. We might then care for one another in more natural, imaginative and wholesome ways: with more sense and sensibility.

*

Men reform a thing by removing the reality from it, and then do not know what to do with the unreality that is left.

G K Chesterton (1928), *Generally Speaking*

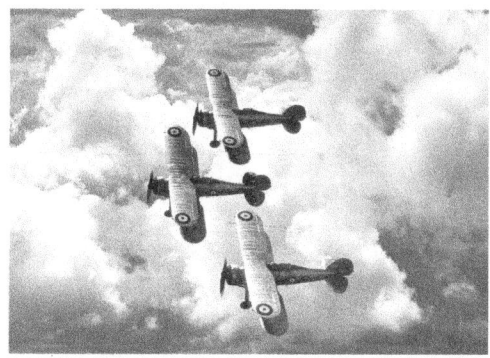

Note

* *Faith, Hope* and *Charity* were the names given to three obsolescent RAF Gloster Gladiator fighter biplanes that were the only aerial defences of Malta at a crucial stage in early World War Two. Due to the skill and heroic resolve of the pilots, these three old planes warded off the vastly more numerous and modern attacking Italian Air Force. Malta occupied a pivotal position for massive opposed forces: the surrender of air-supremacy would have changed world history radically. This remarkable respite created a hiatus sufficient to shift the balance. The full significance of *Faith, Hope* and *Charity* only became clear much later: timely small acts and events can have exponential consequences. Likewise, healing also often needs opportunistic hiatuses into which faith, hope and charity may be both transmitted and take root.

Essay for mental healthcare colleagues and managers South London and Maudsley NHS Trust 2014

Neglect in NHS Healthcare?

We have turned families into factories

The dissolution of family-like configurations in healthcare staffing has impoverished the health and welfare of staff and patients alike.

In December the Daily Telegraph published a letter by eight senior surgeons, which was disturbing in its wider importance (*Surgical teamwork,* 14/12/13). They wrote of how the quality and competence of NHS surgical care has been stymied by successive moves to fragmentation and devolution. Equally significant, they refer to the resulting widespread practitioners' work frustration and dissatisfaction.

Their arguments are pertinent to all areas of NHS healthcare where problems are not simply and speedily resolved: for it is here that personal continuity and investment greatly help accuracy and sensitivity of response. My own areas of practice – as a long-serving GP and Psychiatrist – have witnessed a similar degradation of personally connected and responsible culture.

In their letter the surgeons hark back to now extinct clinical 'firms' which better enacted now-imperilled values: of a personal healthcare ethos. The consultant-led firm, then had its own designated staff, clinic and ward, and was responsible (with rare exceptions) for the total arc of care from initial diagnosis and assessment to surgery, recovery and follow-up. Within this system patients felt more identified, understood and cared for; professional staff shared this, too, in deeper, subtle work satisfactions.

The good surgical firm was like a well functioning family, where the consultant had both directing and nurturing parental functions. This had parallels elsewhere in the NHS: for example, with Medical and Psychiatric firms and the erstwhile small practice family doctor. In all of these, personal investment, responsibility and connection were anchoring professional principles.

In the last two decades – apparently in the interests of mass managed efficiency – we have first not recognised the merits of such 'familial' systems and then pushed them aside in favour of more industrial and commercial modus operandae. We have replaced the spirit of the *family* almost entirely with that of the procedure of the *factory*.

Most veteran doctors of my generation take a similar view to the eight senior surgeons. We see that most of the layers of NHS reorganisation have been expensive follies, both humanly and economically. This is true especially where competition, commissioning and commodification are used to subcontract and devolve. This almost always fragments and depersonalises care.

We have little influence on demographic changes and, maybe, European Working Time directives. But there are other destructive factors we can abolish or substantially revise. Among these are primarily the NHS Internal Market, and then such subordinate devices as autarkic Trusts, Commissioning, payment by results and excessively numerous and boundaried sub-specialties.

Most of healthcare – even surgery – is more of a human interaction than a manufactured commodity. Industry and commerce can only provide very restricted guidance in our complex care of others: Welfare. Our heedlessness of this principle lies behind the broad span of our healthcare malaise: from disgruntled senior surgeons to our Mid Staffs nemesis.

It is the family ethos of Welfare that must command the systems – efficiency of the factory. Not the other way round.

Ω

The Author

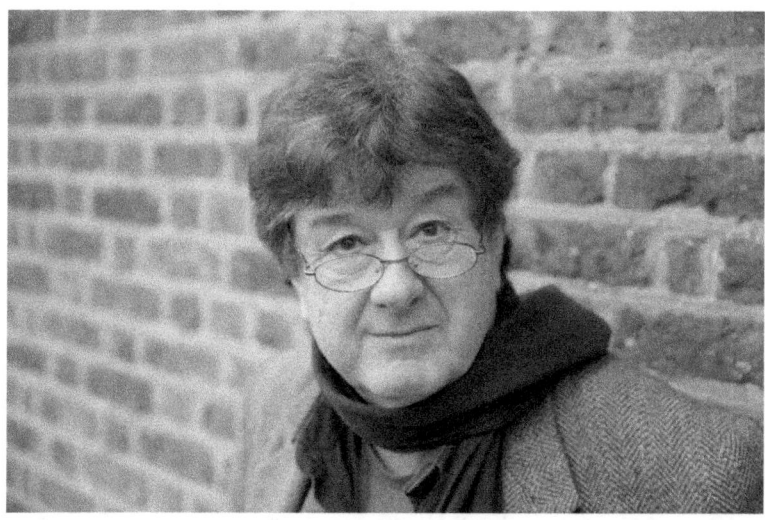

David Zigmond initially trained in Medicine in the 1960s. For several decades he has worked in the NHS as a small-practice GP, and as a large hospital psychiatrist and psychotherapist. Alongside these he has maintained a practice as a private psychotherapist. From these long tenures he has explored the nature and importance of relationships, imagination and personal meaning throughout healthcare. These have fuelled and guided his view and practice of holistic medicine. His long-spanned teaching and writing have been committed to develop and secure these values.

He helped launch the British Holistic Medical Association in the 1980s and has remained active in developing this approach. This book contains many of his contributions.

Other Books on Health
by New Gnosis Publications

Wilberg, Peter *The Illness is the Cure - 2nd extended edition: an introduction to Life Medicine and Life Doctoring - a new existential approach to illness,* 2014

Wilberg, Peter *from Psychosomatics to Soma-Semiotics: Felt Sense and the Sensed Body in Medicine and Psychotherapy,* 2010

Wilberg, Peter *Being and Listening: Counselling, Psychoanalysis and the Ontology of Listening,* 2013

Wilberg, Peter *Heidegger, Medicine and 'Scientific Method': The Unheeded Message of the Zollikon Seminars,* 2012

Wilberg, Peter *Meditation and Mental Health: an introduction to Awareness Based Cognitive Therapy,* 2010

Wilberg, Peter *The Therapist As Listener: Martin Heidegger And The Missing Dimension Of Counselling And Psychotherapy Training* 2008

Zigmond, David *If you want good personal healthcare – See a Vet Industrialised Humanity: Why and how should we care for one another?* (Complete collection, 716 p) 2015

Zigmond, David *The Psycho-ecology of Gladys Parlett – Hidden personal meanings in healthcare* (If you want good personal healthcare – See a Vet, Volume 1) 2015

Zigmond, David *Bureaucratyrannohypoxia* (If you want good personal healthcare – See a Vet, Volume 3) 2015

www.ingramcontent.com/pod-product-compliance
Lightning Source LLC
Chambersburg PA
CBHW051853170526

45168CB00001B/86